MW01286527

To The Point *Series*

Begin As You Mean To Go With

BABYWISE

NIGHTTIME

SLEEP SOLUTIONS

The How and Why of Training Your Baby
To Sleep Through The Night

Gary Ezzo M.A. & Anne Marie Ezzo, R.N.

After a fatiguing and depressing three months of parenting, my sister-in-law handed me a copy of the Ezzo's book. It saved my life! Beforehand, I sought help everywhere: books, friends, experienced mothers, even my baby's pediatrician. I received plenty of advice, but no real solutions that could turn around a 24/7 fussy baby. Seven days after applying the principles, my baby was sleeping 9 hours at night, napping during the day, and his fussiness was isolated to an hour in the late afternoon. The amount of common sense wrapped up in this one book is amazing and very definitely life changing.

A mother from West Covina, California

My husband and I had heard all sorts of horror stories and felt so discouraged and defeated before our baby came. Feeding around the clock, unexplained fussiness, and household chaos was not what we wanted. We were sure there had to be a more sane way to parent than that. We were introduced to the Parent-Directed concepts a week before our son was born. How timely! As predicted, our happy, contented baby was sleeping through the night at eight weeks. We so appreciate the Ezzo's insights, and thank them for giving us the confidence to do what is best for our son.

A mother from Denver, Colorado

Without reservation I would recommend this book to anyone—because it works! I demand-fed my first three children, not knowing there was another way. I did not get a complete night's sleep in five years. When friends began to share your principles, I refused to listen to what I thought was simplistic nonsense. I hold a master's degree in early childhood education, and your concepts challenged everything I had been taught.

When our friends' first child slept through the night at seven weeks, I was enraged. My husband and I watched as their second and third followed the same pattern. They had everything under control, and so few of the problems that we experienced. When I discovered that I was expecting baby number four, I was depressed for months. The only thing I could focus on was the misery of more sleepless nights and demanding children.

I am ashamed to say that it was out of desperation that we applied your parent-directed feeding concepts. I was humbled! Our baby slept through the night at seven weeks. We could not believe it was that easy. He was a delight, happy and content, something never experienced with the first three. Since then, a fifth child has arrived and, again, success. This book has saved our marriage and family. Thank you.

A mother from Philadelphia, Pennsylvania

My husband and I want to thank you for getting us on the right track from the beginning. It was not easy, because all our friends followed the demand-feeding philosophy and said a schedule was bad for the baby. For these families, children were a major interruption. That did not make sense to us. We stayed with your program, and our baby slept 8 hours through the night at six weeks, and 11 hours at twelve weeks—just like your book says. My friends said exactly what you predicted: that we were lucky and had an easy baby. But we know otherwise. Thank you for being a source of encouragement.

A mother from Fort Worth, Texas

I was at church holding a crying baby, and everyone asked what was wrong with my son. They said they had never before heard him cry. Then they realized, I was holding someone else's baby. Thank you for the *Feed - Wake - Sleep* strategy. My wife and I have a happy, contented baby. Before our son was born, we heard so many disturbing stories. My sister had not been out with her husband for three years after the birth of their first son. She went to a mothers' support group but only found other mothers to cry with. No, thank you! Not for my wife. We follow the principles of *PDF*. Because our lives are so predictable, and our son responds so well to routine, we had our first date night after three weeks and once a week ever since. Thank you for helping to keep our family a family.

A father from Tacoma, Washington

Our daughter will be one year old at the end of this month, and I must tell you that I truly and profoundly enjoyed the first year of her life. A big part of the reason is because we followed the sleep training principles presented by the Ezzos. It was not only helpful with my daughter, but it also helped me understand my frustrations with my firstborn! I kept wondering why he was so demanding. Why would he never sleep at night or take decent naps?

I had nursed my son as often as he needed (so I thought)—anytime and anywhere, day and night—until he was 22 months old. And I gave him attention, both quality and quantity. He slept with us at night, but after a few weeks, the baby slept with only me; my husband was sleeping on the couch. I stayed home, gave him a good learning environment, and cooked all natural foods. I did everything the "experts" said to do. But they were so wrong. In the end, it was all for nothing. The only thing I succeeded in doing was to raise a demanding, out-of-control toddler who is not pleasant to be with.

Thank you for your sensible teaching.

A mother from Vancouver, British Columbia

My wife and I were introduced to your program while in marriage counseling. It was then that we discovered the trap of child-centered parenting. In the name of "good parenthood," we gave up our marriage—figuratively and nearly literally. We did this for the "baby's good." That sounded sacrificial and was something I wanted to do as a father. But I never realized how faulty that thinking was until I read your first two chapters. Your book makes sense out of nonsense.

After 18 months of misery, we started our son on a routine. After four nights he began sleeping through the night, and my wife began to sleep with me—but this time alone. What a difference a good night's sleep makes to a toddler's disposition! We had a new son. Get these vital principles out to every family of childbearing age.

A father from Atlanta, Georgia

To The Point *Series* - Book 1

Begin As You Mean To Go With

BABYWISE

NIGHTTIME

SLEEP SOLUTIONS

The How and Why of Training Your Baby
To Sleep Through The Night

Copyright 2024, by Gary & Anne Marie Ezzo

Published By
Charleston Publishing Group

ISBN: 978-1-932740-54-7
Printed in the United States of America

Find us on www.Childwise.Life

Print Run/Year
01/24

Dedicated to:

All those early moms and dads who saw what was possible and shared it with a friend.

ACKNOWLEDGMENTS

According to a host of online dictionaries, the purpose of an "acknowledgment" is to express a debt of gratitude and appreciation to someone who otherwise would not be recognized. These pages exist for that reason. While the cover of this book displays our names as Authors, in truth there were many people from within our community of thought who applied their time, energy and giftedness to help make this book a joint venture for the common good. Most readers will never personally meet these behind-the-scene individuals, but each reader will be the benefactor of their labor.

Where would we be without our medical advisors and friends? We especially wish to thank Dr. Robert Turner for overseeing matters pertaining to pediatric neurology and Doctors Jim Pearson, Stuart Eldridge and Luke Nightingale, who never grew weary with our many questions.

Turning our appreciation closer to home, we are honored to serve with a team of young couples whose collective voices brought a level of clarity to the message that we alone could have never achieved. Among the many are Rich and Julie Young who played an integral role in refining many of the sleep training concepts. Joining the Youngs are Greg and Tara Banks,

To all our contributors, named and unnamed, we say, "Thank you."

Table of Contents

Introduction

*B*abywise Sleep Solutions is a derivative of previous works by the authors, including *Preparation For Parenting* and *On Becoming Babywise.* The need for a condensed version of these successful volumes is in response to a new generation of parents looking for content that gets to the point. Our aim with this new release is to do exactly that—get to the point by keeping the main thing the main thing. In this case, what does it take to help infants learn healthy daytime habits that lead to sleeping through the night? We can explain the critical components of sleep training in a couple of pages, (and will do exactly that), but explaining the broad landscape of parenting will take a more robust level of supplemental knowledge.

The training principles contained in this edition are similar to those in the original books that go back to 1984 when the concepts were first shared. Sarah was the first baby girl raised with the principles; Kenny was the first boy. Both thrived on mother's milk and a basic Parent-directed feeding routine and slept through the night by seven weeks. It was that easy! The positive message continues to spread from friend to friend, city to city, state to state, and country to country. Today, we no longer count the success stories in thousands or even in tens of thousands but in millions of happy, healthy babies who were given the gift of nighttime sleep.

It is our opinion that the achievements of healthy growth, contented babies, good naps, and playful waketimes, as well as the gift of nighttime sleep, are too valuable to be left to chance. They need to be parent-directed and parent-managed. These are attainable conclusions, because infants are born with the capacity to achieve these outcomes and, equally important, the need to achieve them. Our goal is to demonstrate the *how* of nighttime sleep training, and *why* it should be done.

In previous editions of this work, the content unfolded with subjects that extended far beyond the mere mechanics of sleep training. We embraced the entire world of nurturing an infant and caring for Mom. We explored not only the universal themes of the precious first year but also delved into the specific, urgent challenges, such as how to soothe a baby challenged with colic, or find harmony when blessed with multiple births.

Although these rich and varied topics no longer live within these covers, they remain alive, waiting for you to discover them in the virtual realm at *www.Childwise.Life*, under the *Babywise Sleep Solutions* tab. We invite you to wander through these carefully curated, freely offered resources, which have been thoughtfully designed to complement this text. As you move through each chapter, we will point the way to all pertinent resources that are waiting to expand your understanding.

There are some points of language we feel the need to address, small details that carry weight. As you move through the book, you will notice that we often choose to use the masculine gender in our examples. This was a decision of ease, though it is important to say that the principles shared here are universal, just as applicable to girls as to boys. In our desire to speak directly to you, dear reader, we have also used the second person—"you," "your," "yours"—as if we were in conversation with you, face-to-face. You will also find that when we speak of an infant, we simply call him "Baby," that small being who is both specific and universal, unique yet belonging to all.

The principles within these pages are not merely steps to follow but are more like seeds of wisdom, meant to take root in the fertile soil of your family's life. They have bloomed in the homes of millions of parents before you, and with care, they should blossom beautifully for you as well. But please remember, your pediatrician or primary health-care provider is the guardian of your baby's health, and when questions arise, they should be your trusted guide.

Enjoy the journey!

Gary Ezzo & Anne Marie Ezzo
Charleston, SC

Chapter One

The Secret Sauce

To The Point: *The How*

Although training a baby to sleep through the night involves highly complex and well-regulated neuro-biological processes, the actual steps by which these complexities are brought together for successful outcomes are remarkably straightforward. In the following pages, we explain the essential elements that have helped countless parents guide their little ones toward restful nights, adorned with seven to eight hours of continuous sleep by seven to nine weeks of age. Whether your baby is breast-fed or bottle-fed, the outcome remains the same.

The strategy requires adherence to the two guiding principles of feeding. Let's get right to the point.

<u>Principle One</u>: *Feeding during the first 7-10 days*

In these first days, a delicate dance unfolds between mother and child—a time when both find their rhythm, a sacred equilibrium. This is not a period to be enslaved by the ticking of clocks, overly concerned with fixed routines, or the pressures of sleep training. In fact, we encourage you to set aside the concept of time (at least figuratively), focusing instead on the single goal of ensuring your baby receives *full feedings* at each feeding. While a full feeding may not happen at each feed during these early days, the goal remains the same.

For clarity sake, frequent, small feedings do not equate to a full belly, nor do they foster the same satisfying outcome. In fact, they can disrupt a child's ability to connect rhythmic needs with healthy sleep, and that only fosters perpetual sleep disturbances.

Mothers who work in harmony with their babies, ensuring full feedings during these early days, often find their little ones naturally transitioning to a consistent 2½ to 3-hour routine within a week to ten days. Nursing sessions during this period may last between 30 to 40 minutes per feeding, though this can vary—some newborns nurse with speed and efficiency, while others take their time, savoring each moment.

Principle Two: *The symphony of days and nights*

The newborn, so precious, comes into the world like a bud on the verge of blooming, eager to grasp the rhythm of life. As the infant's brain begins a new journey outside the womb, it instinctively seeks to organize and make sense of this new world, yet it is unable to sculpt the cycles of *feed, wake* and *sleep* that are needed to thrive. They need guidance from Mom and Dad.

Like architects and site supervisors, they gently begin building structures within Baby's day. They step in, not with grand gestures but with the small, repetitive acts that will define the newborn's existence. From their consistency, a methodical and predictable feeding routine emerges. Slowly, it becomes more than a feeding routine; it is the foundation of everything that follows—wakefulness, naps, and nighttime sleep.

To secure for your baby peaceable and extended nighttime slumber, this sequence must be held to: *feed, wake,* and *sleep.* There is magic in the order of these steps. Feeding is the beginning, not just of nourishment but of everything—the moment the body starts to settle, preparing itself for the rest that follows. The waking time that comes next is brief at first, a hazy interval between feedings, but as days pass, it stretches, marking the child's gradual awareness of the world. Finally, sleep returns, inevitable and necessary.

This cycle repeats itself, creating a metabolic rhythm, like the rising and falling of the tides, in which all underwater creatures adapt their unique characteristics and needs to the unchanging and ever-predictable ebb and flow. Similarly, the neurological and biological processes necessary for sustained sleep synchronize with the predictable feed-wake-sleep rhythms. Your baby, all the time, learning, adapting, and coming to rely on this rhythm—a rhythm that was initiated from the outside but becomes, over time, internal and natural.

In this early stage of life (during those first seven to ten days) feeding is synonymous with wakefulness. The baby is too new, too small, to do anything more than eat and drift back into sleep. But as the days pass, a subtle shift occurs. A space of time opens up after feeding, a brief but significant period of wakefulness. In these emerging moments of alertness, the baby's consciousness begins to take root, and from here, infantile learning begins. The routine, now set, stretches out across the days and weeks, and life slowly takes shape within its boundaries. This natural progression should reassure parents that they are on the right track leading to the establishment of a healthy feeding routine.

SUMMARY

There you have it—the two guiding principles of infant sleep training. With gentle consistency, the application of the two foundational principles above has been the guiding light for countless mothers and fathers. Forty years ago, we referred to the feed-wake-sleep process as *Parent-Directed Feeding*. Yet, we did not declare it as a new revelation of science, but rather, a name ascribed to the age-old wisdom that has flowed through the hands of our grandmothers from one generation to the next.

These principles, neither rigid nor unyielding, have allowed parents to gift their babies with the serene blessing of seven to eight hours of uninterrupted nighttime slumber. By the time the second moon has passed, parents find themselves standing in the doorway of something they can't quite name, but deep inside they know they have done right by their baby. They have laid down something solid, a foundation that will hold.

HERE COMES THE "HOWEVER"

Yes, the inevitable "however!" Successful parenting is not merely a tally of goals achieved or a checklist of tasks completed but the fruitful vision that comes with *intentionality*. In other words, *begin as you mean to go*. Intentionality is not just about *how* good methods are employed (in this case, sleep training) but also the *why*, which is the profound reason that makes the goal deserving of your attention.

Hear this important truth: No aspect of parenting can be separated from the deeper *why*, for the *why* is the essence that breathes meaning into every decision, whether for the moment or for life. It is the *why* that illuminates the countless benefits that come with achieving our goals.

Now that we have introduced the *how* of infant sleep training, let us delve into the all-important *why*—the heart of the matter—the engine that drives the train.

To The Point: *The Why*

"How did you sleep last night?" is a question that slips out as easily as a sigh, one of those habitual inquiries we often ask those close to us. But have you ever wondered why we do not ask, "How did you greet the morning?" Just as there are differing depths and quality of sleep, there are also different degrees of wakefulness. We know sleep can be peaceful or disturbed, restful or fatiguing. We also know that the quality of our waketime is directly tied to the quality and length of our previous night's sleep. That same truth applies to babies.

Wakefulness also has its range—from a sluggish, drowsy, fatiguing state to one of sharpness and clarity. What truly matters is this single truth: The quality of our sleep directly influences our alertness, which in turn shapes our ability to learn and grow. This connection underscores the profound impact that sleep has on a child's cognitive development.

This connection between sleep and development is particularly significant in the earliest years of life, and specifically during infancy. During the quiet hours of slumber, the brain refines its neural networks, pruning what is unnecessary and strengthening what is essential.

It is a documented fact that babies who sleep soundly through the night are more likely to grow into intelligent children. Unfortunately, so true is the opposite. Healthy sleep habits carried forward from early infancy are so potent they can turn an ordinary child into an active learner, just as quickly as poor sleep habits can nullify a child's full potential. That is because when sleep falters, so does the growth of a child's tender, seeking mind.

This insight is not new; instead, it has been supported by research for nearly a century. Dr. Marc Weissbluth, in his book *Healthy Sleep Habits, Happy Child*, cites the work of Dr. Lewis M. Terman., Dr. Terman is best known for the Stanford-Binet Intelligence Test.[1] Terman's research, first published in 1925, remains influential today. His study of 3,000 children revealed that those with higher intelligence had one thing in common—they all enjoyed consistent, healthy sleep from infancy.

This finding was not a one-time occurrence. In 1983, Canadian researchers replicated Terman's study and concluded that children who sleep well are more likely to have higher IQs. Dr. Weissbluth doesn't just focus on the benefits of good sleep; he also warns of the dangers of poor sleep. When a child's sleep is disrupted, it affects not only their nights but their days as well. They may become less alert, more distracted, unable to concentrate, and physically restless or lethargic.

In the world of infanthood, the failure to establish consistent and continuous nighttime sleep cast long developmental shadows, from dimming the light of learning to increased attachment deficits that show up at six, twelve, eighteen months, and beyond. This is not simple hyperbole. For infants and toddlers, the cumulative consequences of a parenting philosophy that actually suppresses the neuro-biological ability to sleep through the night are particularly serious, for it is only in those precious hours of nighttime slumber that your baby's brain sets about to do its vital work.

A process, known as *myelination* (forming the *myelin sheath*), is the growth of a miraculous covering, a type of lining that insulates and speeds the connections between developing neurons. This amazing neuro activity is switched on during the quiet of the night under cover of restful sleep. That is when the myelin sheath grows, strengthens, and thickens. It initially begins during fetal development and continues into early adulthood. However, it is particularly active during infancy when Baby is experiencing a time of rapid brain growth necessary for healthy development.

We trust the reader can see where we are going here. Sleep, especially continuous nighttime sleep for infants, provides the brain with the optimal conditions for myelination to occur. It is during the long stretches of nighttime sleep that the brain is less focused on processing external stimuli and more on internal processes like cell repair, growth, and myelination. It is the brain's way of building the bridges that will carry a child's present and future thoughts swiftly and surely, enabling and enlarging the connections that define learning.

However, if the good habit of continuous nighttime sleep is never achieved, particularly during this *critical phase* of growth (the period in which a child has the capacity for nighttime sleep but never achieves it), then the brain's work we be continually interrupted. The energy that should nourish myelin sheath growth is diverted, leaving those neural pathways frayed and unfinished. The growth factors that should flow in abundance during sleep, nurturing the brain's delicate architecture, are stifled. And in their absence, the day-brain struggles to keep pace with its own potential. (We encourage the reader to review the intriguing facts related to sleep deprivation in children at *www.Childwise.Life.*)

In summary, healthy infant sleep patterns are integral to the growth and maintenance of the myelin sheath, which is crucial for efficient neural communication and overall brain development. That is the *why*. By providing the brain with the necessary conditions for myelination, sleep ensures that infants develop the cognitive and motor skills needed for a healthy, thriving life. When parents give sleep training the value and honor it deserves, than they are simultaneously embedding within their baby the seeds of tomorrow's success.

TO THE POINT
Having explored the fundamental guiding principles of sleep training

and considered the many benefits that flow from such an achievement, we now shift our focus to the broader world of infant care. It is a certainty that parenting beyond the singular task of sleep training is far more challenging.

The journey is often complex and unpredictable. While there are fixed truths relating to infant development that can guide parents to healthy outcomes, there are also numerous variables that can lead even the most sensible parent into an awaiting labyrinth, containing many intricate passageways and blind alleys. The pages to follow are not merely a supplement to this Chapter, but a type of guiding light that illuminates the many practical, everyday elements associated with the early days of parenthood. They are presented to empower you with the knowledge and skills needed to navigate through the calm and chaos of the unknown and unexpected.

New parents typically have plenty of questions, and that is why we have pulled together a variety of supportive resources that complement this book. Those resources can be found on our interactive website, *www.Childwise.Life*. Becoming child-wise at every developmental phase helps reduce the noise that comes from the burdensome parenting twins *Fear* and *Doubt*.

Chapter Two

Guiding Principles of
Parent-Directed Feeding

One day, sitting by a peaceful pond, I found myself amused by three children, their tiny feet scampering back and forth as they pursued the perfect skipping stone. Who, as a child, has not, at one time or another, tried to skip a stone across the smooth surface of a lake or dropped a pebble in a pool of water and then watched as perfect concentric circles expanded outward from the center? The weight of the pebble breaking the surface creates energy that causes an expansion of ripples, but the initial source that brought this energy to life was the decision to drop the pebble into the water in the first place.

There is a parenting principle tied to this metaphor: Every decision made and every action taken, based on our personal beliefs and assumptions, sets in motion the rippling effects of corresponding outcomes, which are tied to the nature of our beliefs.

Our actions affect the seen and the unseen, often producing unintended consequences. The stone hitting the water, for example, could scare baby turtles floating near the surface, driving them into deep water, possibly toward a predator; the sound of the splash might startle some water birds and cause them to take flight, leaving behind a familiar habitat that provides food and safety. If these collateral actions take place, they are all connected back to us because of a single, momentary decision to throw the pebble in the first place.

RIPPLE EFFECTS OF FEEDING

You would think that establishing good feeding habits would be the easiest part of infant care since a newborn's drive to satisfy hunger is one of the strongest in life. It all sounds fairly simple: Baby is hungry, so you feed him. What more do you need to know? However, the practical side of providing your baby nourishment starts with understanding the interactions between the *constant* influence of time and the *variable* of a child's hunger need..

When it comes to babies, the ripple effect principle is clearly evident in something as basic as how and when to feed a baby. As we will demonstrate in this and other chapters, the feeding philosophy a mother and father decide to implement will produce an ever-expanding series of ripples that impact every aspect of a baby's life. This potential impact underscores the responsibility and attention that parents need to give to their feeding decisions.

That is because, every parenting philosophy has an ascribed pathology and will take parents in different directions and to different outcomes. More specifically, every feeding philosophy is driven by a predetermined set of goals and predefined parenting priorities. Unfortunately, the goals and priorities of the many varied feeding philosophies sound noble and persuasive, but the outcomes are not equal. The more parents understand the components of each feeding philosophy, the better prepared they will be to make an informed decision for their baby's benefit.

INTRODUCING PARENT-DIRECTED FEEDING

While some mothers thrive emotionally on the attachment-style parenting, that is not the case for most women. A more user-friendly, less-fatiguing methodology is called *Parent-Directed Feeding (PDF)*.

The *Parent-Directed Feeding* strategy is the center point between the two extremes—hyper-scheduling and attachment parenting. (The reader can make sense of these titles by reviewing their 20th-century origins. This historical journey of present-day feeding philosophies can be found on *www.Childwise.Life.)* The *Parent Directed* approach has enough structure to bring security and order to a baby's world, yet enough flexibility to give Mom the freedom to respond to any need at any time. It is a proactive style of parenting that helps foster healthy growth and optimal development.

For example, as previously alluded to, a baby cannot maximize learning without experiencing optimal alertness and can only experience optimal alertness with optimal sleep. Optimal sleep is tied to good naps and established night sleep. These advanced levels of sleep are the result of consistent feedings. Consistent feedings are facilitated by a healthy *feed-wake-sleep* routine. *PDF* is the pebble that creates the ripple effect leading to all these outcomes, including measurable parent-child attachment.

Embedded in the parent-directed strategy is the critical element for all aspects of infant care. It is called *Parental Assessment*; an acquired confidence to think, evaluate and intuitively learn what your baby needs and how to meet specific needs at specific times.

What are the advantages of the parent-directed approach? The following comparative analysis of the three common feeding philosophies answers that question and more!

COMPARATIVE ANALYSIS OF FEEDING PHILOSOPHIES
The three prominent feeding philosophies include:

1. *Baby-Led Feeding* (also known as cue feeding, demand feeding, response feeding, ad lib, and self-regulating feeding)

2. *Clock Feeding* (also known as fixed-scheduling)

3. *Parent-Directed Feeding* (*PDF*)

Theories in Practice

Baby-Led Feeding: Feeding times are guided strictly by a single *variable*: the presence of a baby's hunger cues (sucking sounds, hands moving toward the mouth, slight whimpering or crying). The hunger cue is considered a variable because feeding times are random and unpredictable. For example, 3 hours may pass between feedings, then 1 hour, followed by 20 minutes, then 4 hours. It might also be "clusters of feeding," such as five short nursing periods in 3 hours, followed by a long stretch of no feedings. Either way, the time between feedings is not considered essential because the theory insists that parents submit to any cue that looks like hunger, regardless of the lapse of time.

Clock Feeding: Feeding times are guided strictly by the *constant* of time as measured by the clock. The clock determines when and how often a baby is fed, usually on fixed intervals of time. Looking for hunger cues is not considered a priority since feeding times are always predictable. In this way, the clock thinks for the parent and the parent's role is to be submissive to the clock even if Baby is hungry before the pre-determined time to eat.

Parent-Directed Feeding: Both the variable of the hunger cue and the constant of time are viewed as necessary tools of assessment.

THE CONFLICT BETWEEN THE VARIABLE AND CONSTANT
The greatest tension with feeding philosophies tends to center on which feeding indicator to use—the variable of the hunger cue or the constant of the clock. The standard Attachment Parenting doctrine insists on baby-led feedings exclusively. Therefore, the hunger cue is always dominant.

Parents who believe in hyper-scheduling see the fixed segments of time as the final determinant of feeding. Thus, the clock is dominant. The weakness in the logic of these two views becomes obvious when placed into their respective equations. For example, the baby-led equation looks like this:

$$Hunger\ Cue + Nothing = Feeding\ Time$$

"Plus Nothing" in this equation means the presence of a hunger cue is the only consideration that determines when the baby is fed. While this seems to initially make sense, there are some concerns related to this particular approach.

<u>Weakness in practice</u>:
Baby-Led Feeding is based on the faulty assumption that hunger cues, including crying are always reliable. They are not, and that is the primary reason this approach is dangerous. Being guided by the hunger cue only works if a hunger cue, such as crying, is present. Weak, sickly, sluggish, or sleepy babies may not signal for food for 4, 5 or 6 hours and thus, this type of feeding puts the baby at risk of not receiving proper nourishment.

4. Exclusive cue-response feeding can easily lead to infant dehydration, low weight gain, failure to thrive, and frustration for both Baby and Mom.

5. If the hunger cue is consistently less than 2 hours, it leads to maternal fatigue. Fatigue is recognized as the primary reason that mothers give up breastfeeding.[1] They are exhausted!

6. The erratic nature of cluster feeding throughout the day can lead to a range of unintended consequences. These include excessive fussiness, erratic nap behavior, instability in sleep/wake cycles, and all these factors contribute to infant sleep deprivation.

The Clock Feeding equation looks like this:

$$Clock + Nothing = Feeding\ Time$$

"Plus Nothing" in this equation, means nothing but the clock determines when a baby is to be fed.

<u>Weakness in practice</u>:
1. Feeding based on fixed times ignores legitimate hunger cues by assuming each previous feeding was successful. It does not take into account growth spurts, which necessitate a day or more of increased feedings. The baby who shows signs of hunger after 2 hours is put off until the next scheduled feeding, and that extra hour usually comes with crying that could have been avoided.

2.   Strict schedules may not promote sufficient stimulation for breast-milk production, leading to the second most common cause for mothers giving up breastfeeding: low milk supply.

With *Baby-Led Feeding* and *Clock Feeding*, a tension exists between the variable and the constant. This tension is both philosophical and physiological. In either case, as parents are trying to serve their underlying parenting philosophy, they become enslaved to a method. Accepting either of these feeding indicators as an exclusive guide to feeding ensures a stress-filled and, perhaps, unhealthy infant.

PARENT-DIRECTED FEEDING

PDF eliminates the tension of relying exclusively on the unreliable variable of a hunger cue or the insufficient constant of the clock. With *PDF*, both the variable and the constant are used as companions, backups to each other, not antagonists, to be avoided. Consider the *PDF* equation with the inclusion of *Parental Assessment* (PA), which allows Mom to become truly *attuned* to her baby's needs.

The Parent Directed Feeding Equation looks like this:

$$Hunger\ Cue + Clock + PA = Feeding\ Time$$

With the parent-directed approach, you feed your baby when he is hungry, but the clock provides the protective limits so you are not feeding too often, such as every hour, or too little, such as once every 4-5 hours. *PDF* brings into play the critical tool of *Parental Assessment,* which is the ability to assess a baby's needs and respond accordingly. Parental Assessment frees a mother to use the variable of the hunger cue when necessary and the constant of time when appropriate. Here are some of the benefits of the *PDF* approach:

1.   PDF guided by Parental Assessment provides tools to recognize and assess two potential problems with infant feeding:

   •   The breastfed child who nurses so often, such as every hour, may not receive adequate nutrition. In contrast, when using parental assessment, parents respond to the cue by feeding the baby and are alerted to a potential problem with the feeding.

- When the hunger cue is not present, the clock serves as a guide to ensure that too much or too little time does not elapse between feedings. It is also a protective backup for weak and sickly babies who may not always provide tangible hunger cues.

2. When the hunger cue is present, the clock is submissive to the cue because hunger, not the clock, determines feedings.

When Parental Assessment is part of the equation, parents are protected from moving to feeding extremes and their outcomes.

PDF AND MOTHER-CHILD ATTUNEMENT

Attunement is the invisible thread that binds a mother to her child, a connection woven from the delicate tapestry of a baby's unfolding rhythms. And therein lies the key to understanding attunement. It is not merely an instinct; it is the art of listening to the unspoken language, of feeling the vibrations in the air when her child shifts or cries. It is knowing whether the baby's whimper calls for food, for the comfort of a warm embrace, or the serenity of sleep. In these moments, the mother moves in harmony with her child, attending to immediate needs while gently steering the course of their shared journey toward growth.

But this symphony between mother and child is fragile, easily disturbed when there is no rhythm, no routine to give it form. Without the predictable ebb and flow of feeding, wakefulness, and rest, the mother finds herself adrift in a sea of uncertainty, unable to grasp the signals that guide her intuition. Without rhythm there is no melody, just random notes. So it is with attunement.

The essence of attunement sharpens when there is structure, when the melody of the child's routine allows the mother to anticipate, to respond, and to be fully present in the shared rhythm of her baby's life. Without such rhythms, a mother is left navigating the vast and chaotic landscape of unpredictability, where the magic of connection can easily slip away. Too often in the world of baby-led feedings, attunement is reduced to a reactionary response—cry-feed, cry-feed, cry-feed. In the *PDF* world a mother is anticipatory and responsive because there is a rhythm guiding both baby and mom. They dance together in step with a common cadence.

PDF AND INFANT ATTACHMENT

Beyond the assessment tools just presented, the *PDF* principles also facilitate a robust parent-child attachment. This is achieved by creating an orderly environment that allows the baby's growth and development capacities to be optimized. The process is referred to as *attachment cohesion*, a key concept reflecting development's hierarchical nature. It reassures us that the maturation of one group of factors must first be established before subsequent systems can operate correctly. So it is with infant attachment.

The fact that a baby's biological, neurologic and rhythmical needs are merging with his or her natural capacities means nothing is hindering Baby's upward progress toward comprehensive attachment. *"Comprehensive"* refers to the total spectrum of growth and development. If an infant is out of sync developmentally, he or she cannot be in sync with healthy relational or emotional attachments.

Measuring Infant Attachment

"Attachment" is commonly defined by arbitrary "soft" markers that are so broad in scope and futuristic that they have little value when it comes to measuring true infant attachment or exposing attachment deficits. For example, infant attachment is considered achieved if, at some point in the future, a child has healthy self-esteem, good grades, or does not do drugs. As wonderful as these achievements may be, they are too "detached" from infancy to have any relevance. When it comes to babies, true parent/child attachment, must be measured by objective markers relevant to an infant's developmental inclinations. Let's work through this natural unfolding sequence.

The process of attachment has a starting point. It is birth! Contrary to popular attachment theories, the average healthy full-term infant does not enter life burdened with attachment deficits, rather with specific attachment needs. These needs are reflected in capacities yet to be filled. If the fulfillment of these capacities are not made a parenting priority, or if their importance is minimized, the outcomes are predictable. This predictability underscores the need for proactive parenting and can be measured by specific attachment anxiety markers.

In contrast, fulfilling these basic needs provides objective markers confirming the achievement of true attunement and attachment. The healthy markers include babies who:

1. Synchronize their feed-wake-sleep cycles into predictable patterns

2. Can fall asleep without a rocking or nursing props

3. Sleep through the night eight to ten consecutive hours

4. Have a predictable nap routine

5. Have content wake-times and are adept to self-play

6. Are able to self-soothe

7. They are not stressed by Mom's absence but are comfortable with a variety of caregivers (fathers, siblings, grandparents). .

Achievement in these seven areas provides the lead indicators confirming Baby is not stressed or anxious and is at peace with his or her biological, neurological, and relational environment. This is where Mom and Dad's parenting philosophy comes into play. We know a link exists between the absence of these indicators and subsequent pathology of stress. If the attachment-related capacities are stifled or suppressed beyond the timetable of readiness, then the child is forced to adopt coping behaviors, which signal attachment anxiety.

What to Look For

Attachment anxiety is marked by the nine, twelve, eighteen-month, or two-year-old who is not sleeping through the night, not taking regular naps, or cannot nap by him or herself; is unable to self-soothe, is anxious when left alone, or away from mom's physical presence. The baby is not adept at self-play for sustained periods, and nursing is the only form of comfort that can settle the child. In short, these are all lead indicators that the baby's brain is stressed and is existing in survival mode rather than then the growth mode.

The contrasting good news? Each developmental marker that needs to be achieved in order to realize true attachment, are predictable outcomes for *PDF* babies and parents.

Chapter Three

More Facts About Sleep

Imagine a quiet afternoon in a cozy little coffee shop, where you sit with a warm latte, your mind wandering as you browse the web on your mobile device. Nearby, your sweet baby plays contentedly with his bright orange teething ring, occasionally glancing up from his car seat with a serene, trusting gaze. Suddenly, a stranger's kind voice breaks the gentle hum of the café, "Oh my, what a happy baby you have, so content and alert." You return their smile with a nod of appreciation, not surprised by the compliment knowing scenes like this are familiar to parents who follow *Parent-Directed Feeding (PDF)*. What does such a comment have to do with sleep, you might wonder? The answer is everything!

When your baby begins to sleep through the night, people will invariably say, "You're so lucky," or "You've got an easy baby." Neither statement is true. Your baby will be sleeping through the night because you worked diligently to help him achieve nighttime sleep. You deserve credit for your efforts, but keep this fact in perspective: training your baby to sleep through the night is not the final goal of parenting, but it does provide a good foundation on which everything else follows.

Sleep, or the lack thereof, plays a crucial role in a healthy life, especially during the first year when the human growth hormone is released during deep sleep. The quality and quantity of your baby's sleep are vital for their well-being and the entire family's harmony. It's the difference between being a joyful, alert parent or one who struggles through the day, weighed down by fatigue.

New parents who embrace the Parent-Directed Feeding Philosophy can reflect on a legacy of success spanning forty years. *PDF* babies are known for their contentment, healthy growth, and keen alertness. These little ones radiate happiness, a reflection of the restfulness of good sleep. Healthy, full-term babies are born with the potential to achieve 7-8 hours of uninterrupted sleep by seven to ten weeks of age and 10-12 hours by twelve weeks. However, this achievement requires parental guidance and an understanding of how a baby's routine affects development.

Let's review a few facts.

Sleep Fact One:

As noted in Chapter One, the infant brain thrives on predictability and routine! Its natural impulse is to organize. However, newborns do not have the ability to organize their own days and nights into predictable rhythms, even though they have the biological need to do so. That is why parents must take the lead by creating a predictable feeding routine, which gives structure to a baby's day.

Sleep Fact Two:

Also noted in Chapter One is the fact that sleep success is tied to Baby taking full feedings at each feeding. Follow the corollary effect: A good waketime positively impacts healthy naps, and the baby who naps well, is a better feeder. And of course, it is the consistent quality of each of the three activities that eventually facilitates healthy nighttime sleep.

Sleep Fact Three:

From birth onward, infant hunger patterns are pliable, influenced by a routine and, equally, by the lack of routine (results being far less desirable.) When the *Parent-Directed Feeding Plan* guides infants, their hunger patterns stabilize because a baby's hunger mechanism (digestion and absorption) responds to routine feedings with a type of metabolic memory. Bottom line? Routine feedings encourage Baby's hunger metabolism to organize into predictable cycles. Erratic feedings or "clusters of feeding" discourage this.

For example, if a Mom feeds her baby appro
hours—Let's say 7:00 a.m., 10:00 a.m., 1:00 p.m., 4:0(
and 10:00 p.m.—the baby's hunger cycle begins to s)
those times. When that is established, daytime sleep
and then nighttime sleep follows. The exact times above are not as
important as the predictability they represent. There is nothing magical
about those times. Parents can start at 6:00 a.m. if that works better for
them. The principle here is consistency, which leads to predictability.

In contrast, erratic feeding periods work against a child's ability to
organize good feeding rhythms, which creates confusion within the
child's metabolic memory. For example, the Mom who follows a cry-
feeding philosophy may feed him at 8:00 a.m., and 30 minutes later,
when her baby cries, she feeds him again. An hour may pass and he
feeds, followed by 3 hours before the next feeding, then 20 minutes.
The next day, everything is different, including the length and timing
of each feeding cycle. When there is no consistency in the amount of
time between feedings, and when this pattern continues for weeks, it is
very difficult for the feed-wake-sleep cycles to achieve a healthy rhythm.

As a result, these babies have difficulty establishing stable and
uninterrupted nighttime sleep, waking as often as every 2 hours on
a recurring basis. This pattern may continue for two years or more
according to some studies.[1] Not surprisingly, formula-fed babies who
are not on a routine usually end up with the same results.

Sleep Fact Four:
It is not what goes in the mouth as much as when it goes in. Failure
to establish nighttime sleep is not associated with the source of food,
i.e. breastmilk or formula. Our sleep study of 520 infants demonstrated
that *PDF* breastfed babies will sleep through the night on average at the
same rates and, in many cases, slightly sooner than formula-fed babies.
This statistical conclusion means one cannot rightly attribute nighttime sleep to a tummy full of formula. These statistics also demonstrate
that neither the composition of breastmilk or formula nor the speed
at which the two are digested have any bearing on a child's ability to
establish healthy nighttime sleep patterns.

ROMISES, BUT. . .

While we cannot offer any guarantees, we can provide the following statistics that represent *PDF* norms. The following conclusions were drawn from a sampling of 520 infants (266 boys and 254 girls), of which 380 were exclusively breastfed, 59 were exclusively formula-fed, and 81 were fed a combination of breastmilk and formula. There were 468 babies with no medical conditions and 52 with medical conditions detected at birth or shortly after birth. Included in the medical-conditions profile were 15 premature infants. All parents followed the *PDF* strategy.

For the breastfed babies, routine feedings were defined as feeding every 2½-3 hours for the first eight weeks. For the formula-fed babies, routine feedings were every 3-4 hours. Nighttime sleep was defined as sleeping continuously 7-8 hours through the night. Volunteer subjects were drawn from the United States, Canada, and New Zealand. The study revealed the following:

Category One: Exclusively Breastfed Babies

Of the breastfed girls, 86.9 percent were sleeping through the night between seven to nine weeks, and 97 percent were sleeping through the night by 12 weeks of age. Of the breastfed boys, 76.8 percent were sleeping through the night between seven and nine weeks and 96 percent were sleeping through the night by 12 weeks.

Category Two: Exclusively Formula-fed Babies

Of the formula-fed girls, 82.1 percent were sleeping through the night between seven to nine weeks, and 96.4 percent were sleeping through the night by 12 weeks. Of the formula-fed boys, 78.3 percent were sleeping through the night between seven to nine weeks and 95.7 percent were sleeping through the night by 12 weeks.

Category Three: Medical Conditions

Of the 52 infants with medical conditions (e.g., reflux, colic, premature delivery, viral infections, and unspecified hospitalizations), all slept 8-9 hours through the night between 13 and 16 weeks.

As the statistical percentages demonstrate, parents can guide their baby's sleep/wake rhythms quite early and with a high degree of predictability.

BARRIERS TO SUCCESSFUL SLEEP TRAINING

By the time a baby reaches the tender age of two months, there lies within him a natural, almost instinctual capacity to sleep through the night. It's a skill, one that, like all others, thrives on the nourishment of routine. Yet, when sleep eludes them, when their nights become punctuated with restless awakenings, it is a sign that this skill has not yet been activated. The reasons are manifold, but often, the culprits are what we call sleep props—those objects that serve as crutches, helping the baby slip into slumber or return to it when stirred too soon.

Since sleep is a natural function of the body, and its primary cue is the unmistakable sensation of sleepiness. Sleep props interfere with the process by suppressing the innate cue (sleepiness) with an external cue, the prop. No longer does the baby drift off on his own; instead, he becomes dependent, requiring the presence of a parent to offer the prop that has become their ticket to sleep.

Some sleep props, such as a special blanket or a stuffed animal, are harmless, while others can grow into an addictive necessity. Here are a few sleep props to avoid:

Intentionally Nursing Your Baby to Sleep

The scene is all too familiar: A mother, tenderly nursing her infant, feels the slow weight of sleep pulling them both down. She rises carefully, cradling the baby close, moving towards the crib with the utmost caution. Her breath catches in her throat as she lowers the baby down, hoping—praying—that this time, the transition will be smooth. But in that moment of fragile stillness, she is caught between relief and dread, knowing full well that a minor fuss from the baby could mean starting the whole process over again. Who suffers more, she wonders, the mother or the baby? And should nursing be the answer every time sleep is needed? The answer, though painful, is no.

With a gentle yet consistent plan, babies will learn to develop healthy sleep habits. When placed in the crib, they should be awake, no need for the parent to tiptoe or hold their breath. There might be tears or a bit of soft chatter, but in time, the baby will drift off on their own, without the need for intervention. Remember, as a parent, you play a crucial role in this process, and your efforts will lead to a well-rested and content baby.

Motion and Vibration Sleep Props

Modern mechanical sleep props rely on specific stimulation to lull a baby to sleep, either when the baby is first showing signs of tiredness or after the baby wakes prematurely. The most common motion sleep prop is the rocking chair. The question here is not whether you should rock or cuddle your baby. We hope that happens often! But are you using rocking or a variety of dancing motions as sleep props?

Other similar props include the vibrating crib mattress and the baby swing. Some parents have tried the unsafe practice of placing their baby on top of a vibrating clothes dryer. Of course, when all else fails, there is also the nightly drive with baby in the car seat. The sound of the motor and the vibrating chassis of the car sends Baby to dreamland, sometimes. These sleep props work to some extent, but only until the dryer runs out of time, the car runs out of gas, or Mom and Dad run out of patience!

In the short and long run, putting Baby to bed while he is drowsy but still awake facilitates longer and stronger sleep cycles than if placed in the crib already asleep.

Sleeping with Your Baby

Using any of the sleep props just noted may not be the best way to help a child fall asleep and stay asleep, but none of them place a baby at risk. Sleeping with an infant in the same bed does! Since 1997, the American Academy of Pediatrics (AAP), National Institute of Child Health and Human Development, and the U.S. Consumer Product Safety Commission have put out medical alerts warning parents of the death risk associated with sleeping next to an infant and continue to do so year after year. One seven-year study tracked the deaths of over 500 infants due to parents lying next to their babies in such a way that they were partially or totally covering them. Do not be misled by that number; it is a small fraction of actual parental overlay cases occurring each year in the U.S.

The American Academy of Pediatrics public policy statement reads, "There are no scientific studies demonstrating that bed-sharing reduces SIDS [Sudden Infant Death Syndrome]. Conversely, there are studies suggesting that bed-sharing, under certain conditions, may actually increase the risk of SIDS."[2] Further, in 2005 the AAP Task Force on SIDS labeled shared sleep with infants as a "highly controversial" topic, and called the practice of bed sharing as "hazardous."[3] This is why co-sleeping with infants may be the ultimate risk decision of our day, (as it was thirty years ago.) Infant deaths related to unsafe sleeping practices have reached "widespread" proportions; and every one of those deaths was preventable. Infant deaths from SIDS are tragic, but deaths from parental overlay as a result of following a dangerous parenting philosophy are both tragic and needless. Safe and sensible sleeping arrangements start with Baby out of Mom and Dad's bed.

Where Should My Baby Sleep?

Where should the crib or bassinet be located? In the same room with parents, but in a crib or separate room using a monitor? From our forty years of experience, babies who sleep in a separate but nearby room with the aid of a baby monitor tend to sleep through the night sooner than babies who sleep in the same room with their parents

There are advantages and disadvantages to both locations. The benefit of having the baby sleep in the parent's room for the first three or four weeks is limited to convenience for the nighttime feedings. Your newborn will need to be fed at least every three hours, so the closeness of the crib is helpful.

One downside for parents comes with all the unfamiliar sounds and stirring noises babies tend to make. Mothers of newborns are susceptible to baby sounds. These unfamiliar sounds can keep a Mom from falling into her own healthy deep sleep rhythms necessary for her health and well-being. Be sure to check with our health-care provider for the latest AAP sleep updates.

TO THE POINT
The best and safest way to help your little one fall asleep and stay asleep is the natural way. You do not need costly gadgets, a new car, or risky parenting theories. Instead of a sleep prop, confidently establish a basic routine to promote restful sleep.

Feed your baby, rock and love him, but put him down in his own crib before he falls asleep. For more help with night training, look for the additional resources located on *www.Childwise.Life*

Chapter Four

Establishing Your Baby's Routine

We previously defined *Parent-Directed Feeding* as a 24-hour infant management strategy designed to help parents connect with their baby's needs and help baby connect with everyone in the family. The two relevant thoughts within this definition are "24-hour" and "management." The first represents a baby's day and the second speaks to Mom and Dad's involvement in their baby's day—they are to be the managers. But what exactly are parents supposed to manage? The short answer is the continually evolving, changing, and growing needs of their baby.

Children come into this world with basic needs for nutrition, sleep, cognitive growth, love, and security. As a baby grows, these needs do not change, but how they are met will change. Therein lies the challenge. How do you establish a baby's routine that is predictable yet "flexible" enough to meet a baby's growing and changing feed-wake-sleep needs?

Part of the answer comes from understanding the meaning of flexibility. The root word *flexible* means "the ability to bend or be pliable." Think of a rubber band. It can stretch when needed but will return to its original shape. Returning to its original shape is perhaps the most critical element of flexibility. During the crucial early weeks of stabilization, you must shape and form your baby's routine. Too much flexibility will not allow this to happen. That is why a baby's routine must first be established before flexibility is introduced into the Baby's day.

Activities of Your Baby's Routine

In the early days of a baby's life, their routine revolves around three simple activities: feeding, waking, and sleeping. These precious rhythms, with gentle adjustments, continue to guide them through their first year of life. For parents, the challenge lies in recognizing the subtle changes that accompany their baby's growth and knowing how to respond with care and wisdom. To aid in this journey, we introduce the concept of the *Merge Principle*.

THE ART OF MERGING

The term "merge" finds its perfect place in the lexicon of early parenting, for it captures the essence of what must occur throughout the first year of a baby's life. Parental guidance is a delicate art of blending the emerging needs of one stage with those of the next. For instance, while a newborn may begin life with nine or ten cycles of feeding, waking, and sleeping each day, by the time a child reaches ten or twelve months, these cycles have naturally condensed to three feeds, two naps and 10-12 hours of night sleep.

But what becomes of those other eight cycles? They do not simply vanish; rather, they merge, one by one, as the baby grows. The nine cycles gently diminish to eight, eight to seven, and so forth, until the day's rhythm harmonizes into just three distinct moments of nourishment and rest. This natural progression raises several important questions for parents:

1. What changes should be anticipated?

2. When might these changes occur?

3. How should parents adjust to these changes?

Though every child is unique in their timing, there are average milestones when these transitions generally occur. While the earliest weeks and months tend to follow a predictable pattern, the exact moments of change may vary from one child to another. Some babies may start with nine cycles, while others may be comfortable with ten, and still others may find eight to be their natural rhythm. Regardless of these individual variations, the principle of merging remains steadfast. Thankfully, there are timeless guidelines to help parents navigate these transitions with confidence.

Guiding Principles to Merging Feed-Wake-Sleep Cycles

1. *Capacity and Ability*: A mother must always consider her baby's capacity and ability when contemplating any change. For instance, it would be unreasonable to expect a two-week-old to sleep through the night without nourishment, for at this tender age, the baby lacks both the capacity and ability to do so. Thus, it is not yet time to forgo that nighttime feeding.

2. *Time Variation:* As your baby grows, the length of each cycle will naturally begin to vary in length, especially around four months. One cycle might be as brief as two and a half hours, while another stretches to three and a half hours. At six months, the pattern shifts again, reflecting the unique needs of the baby and the hour of the day.

3. *First and Last Feedings*: Regardless of the merging process, the day's first feeding holds strategic importance. Once the baby begins sleeping through the night, the first and last feedings of the day become the pillars around which all other day activities revolve.

4. *Individuality Among Children*: While all babies will experience similar merges, the timing and nature of these changes will differ. One baby may sleep through the night at six weeks, while another may take ten weeks to achieve the same milestone. Yet, by twelve weeks, one may sleep twelve hours, while the other only ten. Each child's journey is uniquely their own.

5. *Two Steps Forward, One Step Back*: The path of merging is seldom linear. While some transitions happen swiftly, most take four to six days to establish a new normal. It is not uncommon for a baby to

sleep five or six hours at night one week, only to revert to shorter stretches before eventually settling into longer, consistent periods of rest.

6. *Breast or Bottle*: These principles apply equally, whether the baby is breastfed or bottle-fed.

FROM PRINCIPLE TO PRACTICE

What signals the time for one cycle to merge into another? In the first year, there are seven significant merges, each marked by a predictable developmental trigger.

Consider what the first two weeks might look like using the sample newborn schedule. There are nine feed-wake-sleep cycles distributed evenly over a 24-hour period. Each cycle, from the beginning of one feeding to the beginning of the next, is approximately 2½ hours in length, which is consistent with an infant's nutrition and sleep needs.

While nine feed-wake-sleep cycles a day sounds fatiguing (and it is), they are also necessary—but only temporary! (The sample times listed on the various schedules found within this chapter are for illustration use only. For example, we are using 7:00 a.m. as the "first morning feed," but realize your baby may start at 6:00 a.m. or 8:00 a.m. or anytime in between. Personalize the times to fit your baby's needs.)

Sample Schedule
Weeks 1-2

1. <u>Early Morning</u>

7:00 a.m.	1. Feeding, diaper change and hygiene care
_____	2. Waketime: minimal
_____	3. Down for a nap

2. <u>Mid-morning</u>

9:30 a.m.	1. Feeding, diaper change and hygiene care, nap
_____	2. Waketime: minimal
_____	3. Down for a nap

3. Afternoon

   12:00 p.m.   1. Feeding, diaper change and hygiene care, nap

   _____   2. Waketime: minimal

   _____   3. Down for a nap

4. Mid-Afternoon

   2:30 p.m.   1. Feeding, diaper change and hygiene care, nap

   _____   2. Waketime: minimal

   _____   3. Down for a nap

5. Late-Afternoon

   5.00 p.m.   1. Feeding, diaper change and hygiene care, nap

   _____   2. Waketime: minimal

   _____   3. Down for a nap

6. Early Evening

   8.00 p.m.   1. Feeding, diaper change and hygiene care, nap

   _____   2. Waketime: minimal

   _____   3. Down for a nap

7. Late Evening

   11:00 p.m.   1. Feeding, diaper change and hygiene care, nap*

* Allow baby to wake up naturally, but do not let him sleep longer than 4 hours continuously at night for the first four weeks.

8. Middle of the Night

   1:00 - 2:30 am 1. Feeding, diaper change, back down.

9. Pre-Morning

   3:30 - 5:00 am 1. Feeding, diaper change, back down.

Now we can consider the *how, when* and *why* of the first merge, which usually takes place between weeks three and six.

The First Merge: Weeks Three to Six

In those early weeks, most babies wake twice at night, perhaps at 2:00 a.m. and again around 5:00 a.m. However, many babies stretch their sleep between weeks three and six, gradually merging these two feedings into a single, middle-of-the-night meal, often around 3:00 a.m. This first merge gently reduces the day's cycles from nine to eight, with the baby now sleeping longer stretches, usually from 11:00 p.m. to 3:00 a.m., and then again until morning.

After this merge, no significant daytime adjustments are needed, although mothers may notice waketimes beginning to lengthen after feeding. Nonetheless, the feed-wake-sleep rhythm remains steady, and the baby's routine becomes a little more predictable each day. Understanding what each merge looks like and when they happen will serve as a guide throughout the first year. Each merge reflects a beautiful journey of growth and change. Your guiding hand in this process is crucial because you are the manager of the merges.

Adjustment to Baby's Routine after This Merge: There are no major adjustments needed to the feed-wake-sleep routine during the day. Mom will notice waketimes are beginning to lengthen, but overall, there is no significant changes. Most babies continue with a 2½ to 3-hour routine.

Sample Schedule

Weeks 3-6

1. Early Morning

    7:00 a.m.   1. Feeding, diaper change and hygiene care,

    _____   2. Waketime: minimal

    _____   3. Down for a nap

2. Mid-morning

    9:30 a.m.   1. Feeding, diaper change and hygiene care

    _____   2. Waketime: minimal

    _____   3. Down for a nap

3. Afternoon

12:00 p.m.	1. Feeding, diaper change and hygiene care
_____	2. Waketime: minimal
_____	3. Down for a nap

4. Mid-Afternoon

2:30 p.m.	1. Feeding, diaper change and hygiene care
_____	2. Waketime: minimal
_____	3. Down for a nap

5. Late-Afternoon

5.00 p.m.	1. Feeding, diaper change and hygiene care
_____	2. Waketime: minimal
_____	3. Down for a nap

6. Early Evening

8.00 p.m.	1. Feeding, diaper change and hygiene care
_____	2. Waketime: minimal
_____	3. Down for a nap

7. Late Evening

| 11:00 p.m. | 1. Feeding, diaper change and hygiene care, nap* |

* Allow baby to wake up naturally, but do not let him sleep longer than 4 hours continuously at night for the first four weeks.

8. Middle of the Night

1:30 - 3:00 am   1. Feeding, diaper change, back to crib.

(Merge Two) Between Weeks Seven and Ten

During the tender weeks between seven and ten, a gentle change often occurs in the routine of many *PDF* infants. Around this time, most

45

babies begin to drop their middle-of-the-night feeding, allowing for a peaceful stretch of eight hours of sleep. As this transition unfolds, the eight cycles of feeding, waking, and sleeping are gracefully reduced to seven. Please note, that while your baby is now slumbering longer at night, he will be taking in less calories, but compensates by taking more nourishment during the day, especially at the first feeding.

You may wonder how long your little one can comfortably sleep before needing to be fed again. A simple guide is this: by five weeks of age, most infants can extend their nighttime sleep by an additional hour for each week of life. Thus, a healthy five-week-old may manage a five-hour stretch, while a baby of seven weeks might sleep contentedly for seven hours.

Adjustments to Baby's Routine After Merge Two: Once your baby merges the middle-of-the-night feeding, some gentle adjustments to the daily routine will be necessary. Before this transition, you likely fed your little one every three hours, which fit neatly into a 24-hour cycle. Now, however, with your baby sleeping through the night, the math requires a bit more thought. Here's how it unfolds: with 24 hours in a day, and eight of those devoted to sleep, you're left with 16 waking hours in which to fit seven feedings. Dividing these hours evenly would suggest a feeding every two and a half hours, which might seem like a step backward.

No mother wishes to feel as though she's regressing in her carefully established routine. Still, there are occasions when feeding more frequently than every two and a half hours becomes necessary. Consider these scenarios:

- Due to busy schedules, many nursing mothers experience a lower milk supply, quantitatively and qualitatively, during the late afternoon feeding (4:00-6:00 p.m.). As a result, she may need to offer the early-evening feeding within 2 hours of the previous feeding.

- Second, growth spurts—those inevitable periods of rapid development—necessitate feeding more frequently than usual.

- Third, when the late evening feeding occurs between 8:30 p.m. and midnight, some mothers feed their babies twice within that window—perhaps at 8:30 p.m. and then again at 10:30 p.m. This practical choice allows the mother to retire for the night a bit earlier without disrupting her baby's precious nighttime sleep.

Now, let us return to the challenge of timing after Merge Two. With 16 waking hours and seven feedings to accommodate, here's our suggestion:

First: *Decide upon the timing of the first-morning feeding.* Will you maintain the original time or establish a new one? Either choice is perfectly acceptable, but a decision must be made. Bear in mind, however, that a later start to the morning feeding may push the late evening feeding closer to midnight—something you might prefer to avoid.

Second,: Once you've settled on the morning feeding time, *schedule the seven feedings* from morning through to the late evening.

Third: *Remember the "first-last" principle.* As you rework your baby's routine, the five remaining feed-wake-sleep cycles must be arranged between the first and last feedings of the day. These cycles need not all be of equal length; indeed, it is likely they will vary. Each mother must find what works best for both her baby and herself, embracing the flexibility required in this delicate dance of nurturing.

As you navigate these early weeks, remember that each adjustment, each careful consideration, is a step toward a more settled and harmonious routine for both you and your beloved child.

Here is a sample schedule after Merge Two takes place.

Sample Schedule After Merge Two
Weeks 7-10

1. <u>Early Morning</u>
    7:00 a.m.   1. Feeding, diaper change and hygiene care

_____   2. Waketime

_____   3. Down for a nap

2. Mid-morning

9:30 a.m.   1. Feeding, diaper change and hygiene care

_____   2. Waketime:

_____   3. Down for a nap

3. Afternoon

12:30 p.m.   1. Feeding, diaper change and hygiene care

_____   2. Waketime

_____   3. Down for a nap

4. Mid-Afternoon

3:30 p.m.   1. Feeding, diaper change and hygiene care

_____   2. Waketime

_____   3. Down for a nap

5. Late-Afternoon

5.30-6:00 p.m.   1. Feeding, diaper change and hygiene care

_____   2. Waketime

_____   3. Down for a nap

6. Early Evening

8:00-8:30 p.m.   1. Feeding, diaper change and hygiene care

_____   2. Waketime

_____   3. Down for a nap

7. Late Evening

10:30-11:00 p.m.   Feeding, diaper change down for the night

(Merge Three) Between Weeks 10 and 15

As your little one continues to grow, you may notice that a new chapter in their sleep routine is beginning to unfold. It is during this tender period, between the tenth and fifteenth weeks, that many *PDF* babies show the ability to drop their late-evening feeding, a milestone that marks their readiness to enjoy a longer, more restful night's sleep. With this gentle transition, seven daily cycles naturally condense into six, allowing your baby to sleep through the night for ten to twelve hours. This range, ten to twelve hours, reflects the unique sleep needs of each child, as individual as the baby themselves.

As this change takes root, you'll find that the morning feeding remains a steadfast anchor in the day's routine. Of course, adjustments can be made for your convenience or the benefit of the family, but the rhythm of the day will now be more predictable. The last feeding of the night will naturally occur ten to twelve hours before the morning feeding, providing a comforting consistency that both you and your baby can rely upon.

For breastfeeding mothers, it is important to stay mindful of your milk supply during this transition. Allowing your baby to sleep for longer than ten hours at night might not provide enough stimulation within twenty-four hours to maintain an abundant milk supply. While this concern may not affect every mother, it is something to consider, especially for those mid-thirty plus moms. It may be beneficial to continue the late-evening feeding, around 10:00 or 11:00 p.m., for the next four to five months. This can provide nourishment and comfort during these precious evening hours, while ensuring a steady supply.

Adjusting Baby's Routine After the Third Merge

With the successful completion of this third merge, assuming your baby is now sleeping soundly for eleven hours at night, with the first feeding of the day at 7:00 a.m. and the last near 8:00 p.m., your daytime routine will naturally adapt. Four additional feedings must be thoughtfully woven into the day, allowing for longer waketimes filled with discovery and delight. Though your baby's naps may not lengthen significantly from the previous phase, the abundant sleep they enjoy at night will ensure they are well-rested and content.

This serene phase will continue until solid foods are introduced, typically around six months of age. As you and your baby navigate these gentle transitions, each new day will bring the quiet satisfaction of a well-established routine that nurtures both baby and mom.

Sample Schedule After Merge Two
Weeks 10-15

1. Early Morning

6:30 a.m.	1. Feeding, diaper change and hygiene care
_____	2. Waketime
_____	3. Down for a nap

2. Mid-morning

9:30 a.m.	1. Feeding, diaper change and hygiene care
_____	2. Waketime:
_____	3. Down for a nap

3. Afternoon

12:30 p.m.	1. Feeding, diaper change and hygiene care
_____	2. Waketime
_____	3. Down for a nap

4. Mid-Afternoon

3:30 p.m.	1. Feeding, diaper change and hygiene care
_____	2. Waketime
_____	3. Down for a nap

5. Late-Afternoon

5.30-6:00 p.m.	1. Feeding, diaper change and hygiene care
_____	2. Waketime
_____	3. Down for a nap

6. Early Evening

| 8:30-9:0 p.m. | 1. Feeding, diaper change down for the night. |

<u>(Merge Four) Between Weeks 16 and 24</u>:

This is when many *PDF* babies begin to extend their morning waketime by merging the early morning feeding and the mid-morning feeding. This merge reduces six feed-wake-sleep cycles to five. As a result, there will be only one feed-wake-sleep cycle between breakfast and lunch (although lunchtime is usually moved up at least a half-hour). This is also close to the time when solid foods might become necessary and can potentially impact the timing of activities within the feed-wake-sleep cycles.

Sample Schedule After Merge Two
Weeks 16-24

1. <u>Early Morning</u>

    _____   1. Feeding, diaper change and hygiene care

    _____   2. Waketime

    _____   3. Down for a nap

2. <u>Late-morning</u>

    _____   1. Feeding, diaper change and hygiene care

  _____   2. Waketime:

    _____   3. Down for a nap

3. <u>Early Afternoon</u>

    _____   1. Feeding, diaper change and hygiene care

    _____   2. Waketime

    _____   3. Down for a nap

4. <u>Late-Afternoon</u>

    _____   1. Feeding, diaper change and hygiene care

    _____   2. Waketime*

    _____   3. Down for a nap

   *   Take note how the late-afternoon waketime activity extends into the early evening, concluding with the bedtime feeding. While there is no naptime between the two feedings in this feed-wake-sleep cycle, a baby may occasionally doze for 30-40 minutes, depending on when the late afternoon cycle began. This is referred to as a "catnap."

5 . Early Evening
  8:30-9:00 p.m.   Liquid Feeding Down for the night.**

** Possible 10:30 or 11:00 p.m. "dream feed" for the breastfeeding Mom.

Note about "Dream Feeds": Mothers often wonder if there is a distinction between the late-evening feeding and what is commonly known as the "dream feed" since both occur around the same time at night. Indeed, there is a difference! The late-evening feeding is a crucial part of your baby's routine, providing the nourishment needed during the first three months of life. The dream feed, however, comes later. It is not given out of necessity, for the baby's calories but rather as a means to help breastfeeding mothers sustain their milk supply. Not every mother will find it necessary to offer a dream feed, but the likelihood increases as a mother reaches her mid-30s.

Merge Five: Between Weeks 24 and 39

As your baby reaches the age of five to seven months, you may observe the beginnings of a delicate transition—one that intertwines the introduction of solid foods with the emergence of what we affectionately call the "catnap." This shorter yet still necessary nap comes into play when your little one no longer requires the full rest of an afternoon nap but isn't quite ready to move straight from a midday slumber to bedtime. Typically occurring in the late afternoon, around dinner time, this catnap can range from thirty minutes to an hour.

While the shift from a full nap to a catnap does not immediately reduce the number of feed-wake-sleep cycles, it gently guides the routine in that direction. It is during this span, between twenty-four and thirty-nine weeks, that most babies make this adjustment, though the timing varies widely from one child to another. Some may embrace the catnap early, while others might hold onto their third nap well into the seventh month. This variation is perfectly normal, a testament to the individuality of each precious child.

Merge Six: Between Weeks 28 and 40

Somewhere within this span of weeks, many *PDF* infants will drop their catnap, further refining their daily routine by reducing the number of feed-wake-sleep cycles from five to four. These four cycles now align with breakfast, lunch, dinner, and a final liquid feeding at bedtime. As with previous transitions, there is a significant variation in timing, which is perfectly natural.

Consider the nighttime sleep patterns of two babies, Cory and Anna. When it came time to drop the catnap, Cory did so at 31 weeks and moved on to Merge Seven. Anna, on the other hand, held onto her catnap until 39 weeks before she was ready to transition. Both babies, though following different paths, were well within the "normal" range for this stage of development, each honoring their own rhythm of growth.

Merge Seven: Between Weeks 46 and 52

As your baby nears the end of their first year, they will reach a significant milestone—no longer needing liquid feeding before bedtime. Whether it's a cup of formula, breastmilk, or water the days of a bedtime bottle or nursing will soon be a fond memory. Congratulations, dear mother, for you have journeyed far from those early days of nine feed-wake-sleep cycles, navigating each transition with grace and care.

Though we have walked through a year's worth of transitions, let us now turn our attention back to the early weeks, those precious first twelve weeks of your baby's life, where the foundation of feeding, waketime, and naptime is lovingly laid.

SPECIFIC FEEDING AND WAKETIME GUIDELINES

Although we just surveyed a year's worth of transitions, this next section returns the reader to the first twelve weeks of a baby's life and offers specific reminders related to feedings, waketimes and nap times.

Feeding and the First Twelve Weeks

<u>One</u>: During the first week, newborns are sleepy and sleepy babies are prone to snacking: a little food now, a little food later. A series of snack feedings do not add up to full feedings. Baby needs to eat, and the breastfeeding mom needs the stimulation that comes with full feedings.

<u>Two</u>: For a newborn, the duration of time awake, including feeding, burping, diaper change, cuddles and kisses, will be approximately 30 minutes. Sleep follows the feeding and that takes up the next 1½ to 2-hours. When adding it all together, the entire feed-wake-sleep cycle averages 2½-hours until the cycle repeats itself.

<u>Three</u>: Around the third week postpartum, your baby will begin to extend his waketime after each feeding. This time will eventually extend to thirty minutes beyond feeding. On average, waketime is followed by a 1½ to 2-hour nap.

<u>Four</u>: At six weeks of age, feeding times are still approximately 30 minutes and waketimes begin to increase to 30-50 minutes, followed by a 1½ to 2-hour nap. By twelve weeks, waketimes could be a full 60 minutes or slightly more.

How to Merge or Drop Feedings

Babies "drop feedings" because they are either sleeping longer or staying awake longer. As a reminder, the act of "dropping a feeding" is part of the larger merging process and requires adjustments to the baby's daily routine. On paper, we can make everything work out, but babies often need some help. This is where the collective wisdom of experienced mothers comes in handy. Here are a few time-tested suggestions to consider.

1. Dropping the middle-of-the-night feeding:

Between weeks seven and ten, most *PDF* babies drop the middle-of-the-night feeding on their own. One night, they simply sleep until morning. Other babies gradually stretch the duration between the late-evening feeding (10:30 p.m. to 11:00 p.m.) and the first middle-of-the-night feeding until it becomes the morning feeding.

However, there will be occasions when Mom is on board with the idea of an eight-hour sleep and desires to make the adjustment, but Baby is not a willing partner. He has the capacity and the ability, but sometimes may need a little nudge because his internal sleep-wake "clock" is stuck. You will know this is the case if he is waking within five minutes of the same time each night for three consecutive nights.

There are a few ways to handle this. One is to allow the baby to resettle himself without Mom or Dad's direct intervention, or at a minimum, offer a gentle pat on the back to let him know you are there, Normally, after three to four nights with some restlessness, the sleep-wake clock adjusts, and Baby begins sleeping through to morning.

A second method is for Mom to push the late-evening feeding closer to 11:00 p.m. or midnight. Once Baby is sleeping through to the first-morning feeding, she can gradually push the late-evening feeding back by 15-30 minute increments until the feeding time is what she is seeking. A third method, called the backward slide, is a last resort. This is how it works: If your baby is consistently waking at 2:00 a.m. each night, preempt this nightly ritual by waking and feeding him 15-30 minutes earlier—around 1:30 a.m. If he sleeps to his normal morning waketime, in a couple of days, try moving the time back by half an hour to 1:00 a.m.

You can continue this backward slide until your baby's late-night feeding is at a time you are comfortable with. The way you know you are making progress is if your baby is sleeping from the end of this earlier feeding to the first feeding of the day. When you are working to establish a new sleep routine for your baby, stick with it. You and your baby will arrive at your goal and you both will be better off when it happens.

2. Dropping the late-evening feeding:
This occurs around three months and is usually the trickiest feeding to eliminate. Having grown accustomed to sleeping all night, some

parents are reluctant to drop the late-evening feeding for fear that the baby will wake in the middle of the night. If your baby is showing a lack of interest or is difficult to awaken for this feeding, those are good indicators that he's ready to drop it.

The way to drop this feeding is by gradually adjusting the other feeding times. For example, if the late-afternoon feeding is around 6:00 p.m., try feeding the baby again at 9:30 p.m. for a couple of days. Then, move the feeding to 9:15 or 9:00 p.m. for the next two or three days. Continue gradually adjusting the time backward until you reach your desired time for the baby to go down for the night. Dropping the late-evening feeding will often make the last two feedings less than 3 hours apart. That should not be a problem providing the last feeding of the day is the priority.

Sleep Guidelines and the First Month

Waking a sleeping baby for food: If you need to awaken your baby during the day to prevent him from sleeping longer than the three-hour cycle, do so. Such parental intervention is necessary to help stabilize the baby's digestive metabolism and help him organize his sleep patterns into a predictable routine. The one exception to waking a sleeping baby comes with the late-evening and middle-of-the-night feedings. During the first month a baby may give Mom and Dad a 4-hour stretch at night. However, do not let the baby sleep longer than 4 hours. Wake your baby, feed him and put him right back down to sleep. An infant under four weeks of age is too young to go much longer without food.

Waketime and the First Three Months

During the first two weeks of life, your baby will not have a distinct waketime apart from his feeding time. Your baby's feeding time *is his* waketime, because that is all a newborn can handle before sleep overtakes his little body again. Usually by weeks two or three, most babies fall into a predictable feed-wake-sleep routine. When this happens, you and your baby have reached another level of success.

Once you make it through those first couple of weeks filled with new experiences, life begins to settle in as your baby's routine takes shape. What might a feed-wake-sleep routine look like in the first two weeks of your baby's life?

Birth to Two Weeks

Feeding Time / Waketime	Sleep
30-50 minutes	1½ - 2 hours
├─────────── 2 to 3 hours ───────────┤	

In the diagram above, please note the light gray-tone of waketime. It reflects the fact that during the first week, feeding time is basically a baby's waketime. The 30 to 50 minutes noted include feeding, diaper change, burping, and any other hygiene care necessary, not to mention cuddles and kisses. Sleep normally follows feeding, and that should take the next 1½ to 2 hours. So, the entire feed-wake-sleep cycle will range between 2 and 3 hours, before the cycle starts over.

Now note the slight change in weeks three through five.

Three to Five Weeks

Feeding Time	Waketime	Sleep
30-60 minutes		1½ - 2 hours
├─────────── 2½ to 3 hours ───────────┤		

Around week three, you will notice that waketimes are starting to separate as a distinct activity and may last up to 30 minutes. We are not saying your baby's waketime will be 30 minutes; rather, it may last up to 30 minutes in addition to feeding time. Waketime is usually followed by a 1½ to 2-hour nap. With healthy sleep habits established, accompanied by longer waketimes, a new level of alertness begins to emerge that requires additional thought and planning.

Moving to week six, your baby's waketimes become very distinct, and the length of feeding time more precise.

Six to Twelve Weeks

Feeding Time	Waketime	Sleep
30 minutes	30-50 minutes	1½ - 2 hours
├─────────── 2½ to 3½ hours ───────────┤		

Waketimes are followed by the typical 1½ to 2-hour nap, depending on your baby's sleep needs. By week 12, waketimes could be 60 minutes or longer. By then, your baby should be sleeping through the night, so you will offer one less feeding in a 24-hour period.

However, as waketimes begin to lengthen, there is the potential for a subtle and undesired shift in Baby's feed-wake-sleep routine that must be avoided at all cost. Do not allow a "wake-feed-sleep" order to overtake the established "feed-wake-sleep" routine. Here is how this subtle shift occurs. Mom is feeding her seven-week-old, but today, Baby falls asleep without an adequate waketime. After a shorter-than-normal nap, Baby wakes but is not interested in feeding because he is not hungry. Trying to keep Baby on schedule, Mom then holds off the feeding for twenty to thirty minutes. Instead of feeding after his nap, when he is well rested, Baby is now feeding after waking time when he has less energy to feed efficiently.

It is not a big deal if this happens once or twice. However, if this subtle shift continues to repeat itself off and on, even for a couple of days, then Baby's routine will begin to reflect a "wake-feed-sleep" cycle. Here is the problem with that routine. Inadequate waketimes lead to insufficient sleep, resulting in shorter naptimes; shorter naps lead to inefficient feedings, and from there, everything falls apart. That is why feedings, in the early months, should follow after naps and not waketimes.

SOME GENERAL GUIDELINES: CONSIDERING CONTEXT
Context! Understanding the practical implications of this word will prove to be a valuable tool throughout your parenting. Looking into the context of the moment allows you to make a decision based on what is best, given the present circumstances. Responding to the context of a situation allows a mother or father to focus on the right response in the short term without compromising long-term objectives. Here are some examples of context and *PDF* flexibility:

1. The two-week-old was sleeping contentedly until his older brother decided to make a social call. Big brother notifies Mom that Baby

is awake and crying. It is another 30 minutes before his next scheduled feeding, so what should she do? She can try re-settling the baby by patting him on the back or holding him. Placing him in his bouncy seat is a second option, and a third is to feed him and rework the next feed-wake-sleep cycle. Be sure to instruct the older brother to check with Mom before visiting his sleeping sibling.

2. You are on an airplane, and your infant daughter begins to fuss loudly. The mental conflict begins; she just ate a little over an hour ago. What should you do? The solution is to consider the preciousness of others. Do not allow your baby's routine to override being thoughtful to others. If all attempts to play with and entertain the baby fail, go ahead and feed her, for the context of the situation dictates the suspension of your normal routine. Once you arrive at your destination, make the appropriate adjustments to your baby's schedule. There is your flexibility!

3. You just fed your son before dropping him off at the church nursery and are planning to return within an hour and a half. Should you leave a bottle of breastmilk or formula, just in case? Yes, most definitely! Nursery workers (and baby sitters) provide a valuable service to parents. Because their care extends to other children, they should not be obligated to follow your routine to the minute. If your baby fusses, the caretaker should have the option of offering a bottle. Receiving early feedings a few times a week will not ruin a little one's well-established routine.

4. You have been driving for 4 hours and it is your daughter's normal feeding time, but she is asleep and you only have another 40 minutes to travel. You may choose to pull over and feed your baby, or you may just wait until you arrive at your destination and adjust the next feed-wake-sleep cycle.

Most days will be fairly routine and predictable, but there will be times when flexibility is needed due to unusual or unexpected circumstances. Life will be less tense when parents consider the context of a situation and respond appropriately for the benefit of everyone. Thoughtful parental responses often determine whether a child is a blessing to others or a source of mild irritation.

TO THE POINT

The way you respond to your baby's needs—whether it's feeding, waking, or sleeping—reveals much about the kind of parent you are becoming. There is a language in these daily rhythms, a quiet dialogue between you and your child that speaks to your attentiveness and care. Establishing a routine and knowing when to adapt it as your baby grows is not just about managing time; it's about being attuned to the subtle shifts in your baby's world.

At the core of the *Parent-Directed Feeding* strategy lie three simple yet profound activities: feeding, wakefulness, and sleep. Each action is a thread in the fabric of your baby's early life, woven together with your love and intention. By aligning your care with their needs, you guide them through these first months, not just with a sense of duty but with confidence and grace. In doing so, you lay down the first stones on the path of their lifelong well-being.

As you move forward, the next chapter will expand on this foundation, exploring the nuances of extended wake times, the importance of maintaining healthy nap rhythms.

Chapter Five

Waketimes And Naps

As your baby moves from the early days of infancy to the mid-year mark, subtle growth shifts continually influence the various daytime feed-wake-sleep cycles. These small but significant growth changes are challenging to measure in any one moment, but they are present, working behind the scenes, propelling Baby forward. Parents may not visually notice the changes day to day, but they are influencing those changes, especially during Baby's waketimes.

During the early months of life, the activities during waking hours should be seen in terms of a baby's developing mind and their need for proper sensory stimulation. While awake times should involve interaction between Mom, Dad, and Baby, there should also be times when Baby is alone, completely absorbed in their own world of discovery. Healthy nap patterns are closely related to wake times.

We will take up naps and nap challenges in the second half of this chapter, but before we put the little one down to sleep, let's talk through the various activities that should be part of your baby's waketimes.

MOM, DAD AND BABY

Feeding: Whether the liquid nourishment is formula or breastmilk, Mom will hold her baby while she feeds him. Please take advantage of these routine opportunities to gaze into his eyes, talk to him, and gently stroke his arms, head, and face. Touch is essential because it is the first language that newborns need and crave. Babies come into this world with a powerful need to be touched, held and cuddled. Being held communicates security, that their new world in Mom and Dad's arems is a safe one. To fully understand the power of human touch please visit the "Book & Download" page on the *Childwise* website.

While they do not need to be held 24/7 or have constant skin-to-skin contact with Mom, they do need to be held by the many members of their loving community, including Dad, brothers, sisters, and grandparents. The more hands communicate love through touch, the more secure the child.

Singing:
A baby will respond to his mom and dad's voices shortly after birth. During waketimes, parents should enjoy talking and singing to their babies, remembering that learning is always occurring. The simple "la la la la la" sound of his parents' voices will have relational meaning to a baby, even though the words do not. Children memorize words more quickly when they can sing them. That means it is never too early to start working with your child to teach him how words can be used.

Reading:
Likewise, it is never too early to read to your baby or to show him colorful picture books (especially cloth, plastic, and other durable books that the baby can explore on his own). Your little one will love to hear the sound and inflections of your voice.

Bath Time:
This is another pleasant routine for your baby. Mom or Dad can sing, talk, and share their inner thoughts, or just have fun splashing and making the baby's rubber duck quack! (The reader will find many helpful safety tips at the *www.Childwise.Life* resource center.)

Playing:
While smiling, cooing, and little giggles are all part of baby play, the best part of a baby's waketime is when he gets to cuddle with Mommy, Daddy, siblings, or his grandparents. Such feelings of love and security cannot be replaced. .

Walking:
Your baby cannot walk, but Mom and Dad can! Going for a stroller ride and getting some fresh air is great fun for Baby, and walking is great exercise for Mom and Dad. Strollers that have the Baby facing outward provide a more significant opportunity for learning because he can see the world around him. His brain takes in new sights, sounds, colors, and the beauty of nature.

Another option is double-strap, front-pouch baby carriers. They come in various styles, shapes, colors, and fabrics and are easy ways to take Babies on walks, hikes, or strolls through a store. Look for one that fully supports your baby through his thighs, bottom, and back and distributes his weight evenly to your hips while being supported by both shoulders.

Baby Playtime:
When young mothers gather to talk and show off their new little ones, it is common to hear differing opinions on many topics, including how best to manage a baby's day. Planning some alone time into a baby's day is a topic that evokes a variety of opinions. Most parents with an infant in the home tend not to think about this, yet some monitored alone time provides critical learning opportunities. By "alone," we do not mean leaving the baby out of sight but instead providing opportunities for him to investigate his world without being constantly entertained. How can a mom make this happen? Experienced *PDF* Moms will tell you it is a gradual process starting with something as basic as the infant seat.

Infant Seat:
This is one piece of practical baby equipment that is especially handy during the first few months of a baby's life. For clarity's sake, the term "infant seat" is now equated with an infant car seat. However, we are speaking of a portable infant seat that elevates Baby just enough to view his little world. Parents can find a place for the infant seat just about anywhere. In the early days, the swaddled baby can take a nap in the infant seat. As he becomes more alert, he can join Mom and Dad at mealtimes or be placed in front of glass door to view the outside world.

The Bouncy Seat:

This seat is designed for the baby who can hold his head upright without support, usually at three to four months. It is easy to move wherever Mom or Dad may be. If Mom is in the kitchen, the baby can watch her prepare dinner. If she is folding laundry, the baby is happy to watch this activity and keep her company. The bouncy seat is also great for babies who struggle with a mild form of reflux. Keeping the baby upright 10-15 minutes after each feeding helps her food to settle and minimizes spitting up. Be sure to fasten the safety straps, and never leave your baby unattended. As with all baby equipment, take the time to read the safety instructions.

Mobiles and Crib Gyms:

Moving and musical mobiles help a baby learn to track with his eyes, but first he must be able to focus. Since that takes place about three to four months after birth, hold off until then before introducing a crib mobile. Crib gyms and objects that dangle over a baby and rattle when he bats at them help to develop his hand-eye coordination. Batting is the necessary preparation for a baby to reach out and hold objects in his hands. For safety's sake, do not place a crib gym or mobile over a baby once he learns to sit up and grab.

Playpen:

Once parents have their infant's feeding and sleeping routine under control, it's time to work on waketime activities. One essential piece of equipment that will help facilitate waketimes will be the pack-and-play or the playpen. Playpen use will become more common once the baby becomes mobile and can sit up by himself. Here are a few benefits of the playpen.

1. It provides a safe environment. When Mom's attention must be elsewhere and it's not the Baby's naptime, the playpen is about the safest place in the house he could be, other than his crib. This allows Mom to take a shower care for her other children, and do a host of other activities knowing her baby is safe.

2. It doubles as a portable bed. Using the paypen as a bed is especially useful when taking a trip or visiting another home. The playpen gives the baby a clean and familiar place to sleep.

3. It offers a structured learning center. Your baby's first structured learning takes place in the playpen. The partnership a child has with the playpen helps establish foundational intellectual skills. Having playpen time every day allows a little one the opportunity to develop the following:

- Mental focusing skills (the ability to concentrate on an object or activity at hand and not be constantly distracted.)
- A sustained attention span
- Creativity which is the product of boundaries, not freedom. With absolute freedom, there is no need for creative thinking or problem solving.
- The ability to entertain himself
- Orderliness

Parents can begin using the playpen as a portable bed soon after the baby is born, and for tummy time, once the baby has some sustained waketime, he can hold his head up and can explore an item in his hands. The more significant benefit of the playpen begins once a baby can sit up by himself. That is when the playpen should become a routine part of a baby's day.

Whether used for tummy time or later on for a learning center, playpen advantages are only gained if a baby is fresh and alert when using it. Putting a baby in a playpen just before naptime will encourage fussiness, not learning. Parents can begin with ten to fifteen-minute increments of time and gradually extend the time to thirty or forty minutes. Keep several interesting toys within your baby's reach, including one of his favorites. The internet is a good resource for age-appropriate toys and activities. We do offer one word of caution. Do not overload the playpen with too many toys. This works against a child's ability to sit, focus, and concentrate. Three or four toys are sufficient at any one time. Too many toy choices too early works against a child's developing sense of concentration.

Pictures:
All babies are born extremely nearsighted, which means they have difficulty focusing on objects at a distance. That picture hanging on the wall six feet away is quite blurry to your newborn. As each week passes, your baby's eyesight gradually improves and becomes typically 20/20 by the time he is two. You may want to wait three or four months before adding bright, colorful pictures to the nursery decor.

Swing:
Infant swings have evolved significantly since the Ezzo family purchased their first one over fifty years ago. In those days, swings had one purpose: gentle back-and-forth motion. Today, these swings offer a wide range of features, from multiple speeds to various reclining positions, and even soothing music to accompany the rocking. The reclining option is especially helpful after feeding, as it eases the pressure on a baby's full stomach. While the swing gives your little one a chance to observe their surroundings, it's important not to rely on it for naps. For fussy babies, a stronger rocking motion often helps them settle, while a slower speed is ideal for more peaceful, content moments.

Tummy Time:
For those familiar with the author's pioneering work on this specific topic, "Tummy Time" became a successful counter-measure strategy to correct the deficiencies created by the 1992 SIDS "Back to Sleep" campaign, which required babies to sleep on their backs instead of their tummies. As a result of that campaign, pediatricians and family care practitioners began to notice a significant increase in *plagiocephaly*, which is the medical term for the flattening of the baby's head. Also recorded were delays in strengthening the neck and leg muscles necessary for lifting the head, rolling over and crawling, as well as delays in fine motor skills and ultimately cognitive skills.

Fast forward twenty-plus years. Today, the American Academy of Pediatricians, The World Health Organization and the National Institute of Health publicly recognize the long-term value of "tummy time training." Although the organizations above suggest starting Tummy Time training soon after birth, we recommend parents begin after the first month. Our recommendations based on the fact that newborns do not have an extended waketime. In fact, let us remind your that a newborn's feeding time is his waketime. It is only after week four that infant waketimes stretch sufficiently to allow parents to initiate meaningful Tummy Time training.

One of Baby's favorite places to have tummy time is on Mom or Dad's chest. Gently move your baby's arms while talking to him and smiling at him. While you are engaging your baby, he is responding by lifting his head and looking at you. Having tummy time on a blanket as part of the baby's routine can begin once the baby can lift his head, even if only for a second or two. Eventually, tummy time will be the baby lying on a blanket or in a playpen for a sustained period investigating a toy or the bright-colored teething ring.

Regardless of age, the ideal time to have tummy time is shortly after feeding, while he is alert and happy, but not before a nap when he is tired and may fall asleep. Tummy time is a waketime activity you can easily plan into your baby's routine. A minimum of thirty minutes of tummy time spread over the course of the day will help to optimize your baby's healthy growth.

Finally, we offer this note of clarification and caution. Tummy time training does not mean parents should disregard the AAP warnings about baby napping on his tummy and SIDS. The Academy still recommends infants sleep on their backs for at least one year of age. However, this may not be practical since babies can roll over onto their tummies by seven to nine months.

NAPTIMES AND BASIC SLEEP NEEDS

Adequate sleep is essential to a baby's life and will continue to be beyond his first year. Newborns will nap frequently. While parents will not be actively involved in sleep training before four weeks of age, they will do so passively by establishing an excellent feed-wake-sleep routine. The next couple of pages contain nap/waketime summaries highlighting what parents can expect throughout the first year.

Newborn

Newborns can sleep 17-19 hours per day, including the sleep periods between each feeding. With *PDF*, this sleep will come in five to six naps (depending on the number of daily feedings). After feeding, when your baby has been up for an appropriate duration and begins to show signs of sleepiness, such as rubbing his eyes, yawning or tugging on his hair, it is time to go back down for a nap.

One to Two Months

By week four, waketime emerges as a distinct activity; by eight weeks, it is fully developed. The average nap for a two-month-old is 1½ hours long, with some naps a little longer and some a little shorter. At the end of this period, 75-80 percent of *PDF* babies drop their nighttime feeding and begin sleeping 7-8 hours continuously through the night. Continuous nighttime sleep will follow for the remaining 20 percent in a couple of weeks.

Three to Five Months

At three months, the length of the baby's naps fluctuates a bit. Most naps fall between 1½ to 2 hours. During this growth phase, Baby may start waking earlier in the morning and begin to take shorter naps during the day. By five months, the average *PDF* baby takes two 1½ to 2-hour naps and an additional late-afternoon catnap daily.

Six to Eight Months

Between six and eight months, parents will find their baby's daytime sleep needs decreasing as his waketime increases. By this time, the late-evening feeding has been dropped, leaving four to six feeding periods during the day. Nighttime sleep will average 10-12 hours. The baby will have two daytime naps between 1½ to 2 hours in length and possibly a catnap. Once the catnap is dropped, both waketime and often the other remaining naptimes will increase in duration.

TO THE POINT: NAPTIME RESOURCES

We wish not to be the barer of bad news, but the serene slumber you so carefully nurtured in the early weeks will eventually falls under the influence of nap disruptions and daytime sleep intruders. The reasons are multiple, and can be very challenging.

To whom can a mother turn when seeking the guidance needed to restore peace to her baby's naps? Take heart. We have anticipated these challenges and have responded with careful and clear guidance available on our resource page at *www.Childwise.Life.* There, the weary mother will discover a wealth of articles and explanations that might seem like they were penned with her struggles in mind. There are numerous nap disturbance scenarios presented along with solutions, and if you like, a friendly voice that can help you sort things out.

The *Nap and Naptime* resource page will soon become a trusted companion, offering solace and solutions to the perplexing disruptions that may suddenly besiege a well-established nap routine. Though formidable, these challenges are not insurmountable, and there is abundant help awaiting those parents who earnestly seek it. With the right resources, you will find the strength and knowledge to overcome these obstacles and restore your child's peaceful slumber.

Chapter Six

The How of Nourishment

The tender beginnings of a baby's life are best adorned with an abundance of cuddles, kisses, and the gentle care of proper nourishment. While the former comes naturally to the loving parent, the latter requires a bit more understanding and thought. Whether a child receives nourishment from the breast or from the bottle, the most essential ingredient is the affection and attention with which the feeding is given.

There are differences between these two sources of sustenance and, understanding them will help new parents feel assured in making the best decision for their baby and their family. What facts should expectant mothers and fathers consider?

First and foremost, feeding a baby is one of the most fundamental acts of care. A newborn's reflexes for sucking and rooting are well-developed, and the little one will naturally seek to satisfy them by turning toward anything near its mouth. In the grand comparison between breastmilk and formula, it is hardly surprising that a mother's milk is often hailed as the ideal nourishment, offering numerous benefits that promote health and well-being.

The American Academy of Pediatrics tells us that research suggests breastmilk may decrease the incidence or severity of common ailments such as diarrhea and lower respiratory infections, as well as more severe conditions like bacterial meningitis and urinary tract infections.[1] Moreover, breastmilk is believed to provide protection against Sudden Infant Death Syndrome, allergic diseases, and certain chronic digestive issues.[2] It is easily digested, perfectly balanced in nutrients, and rich in antibodies that help build a baby's immune system. There are likely even more benefits to be discovered in this wondrous natural provision.

Unlike formula, which requires some preparation and warming, breastmilk is always ready, always fresh, and never in danger of spoiling. There are also considerable benefits for the mother. Breastfeeding aids in the uterus's return to its normal size, and it can help with postpartum weight loss; a joyful benefit for any mother eager to return to her pre-pregnancy wardrobe. Additionally, recent studies suggest that breastfeeding may lower a mother's risk of developing breast cancer, Type 2 diabetes, and osteoporosis later in life.

HUNGER CUES

A mother's prompt response to her newborn's hunger cues is key to successful feeding, whether she follows a cry-feeding or a parent-directed feeding (*PDF*) approach. The *PDF* method encourages full feedings every two and a half to three hours rather than a series of small, scattered snacks. As we learned in Chapter Two, achieving full feedings is crucial to the success of this method.

"Listen to your baby's cues" is indeed wise advice, but it requires that parents know what to look and listen for. As a baby nears the end of a sleep cycle, you may notice soft sucking sounds or see the little one bringing a hand to the mouth, followed by a gentle whimper that may escalate to a full cry. These are signs that it's time to eat, but there's no need to wait until the baby is in full cry before responding. The hunger cue should always take precedence over the clock.

However, not all cues are welcome. If a baby is nursing every hour, it might be a sign that the little one isn't getting enough of the rich, high-calorie hindmilk, or that proper sleep is lacking. Remember, a well-rested baby is more likely to nurse well, and good sleep promotes healthy growth. A mother who wakes up every morning feeling exhausted from multiple night feedings should take this as a sign that her routine might need adjusting.

MILK PRODUCTION AND FULL FEEDINGS

If you choose to breastfeed, there are some basic principles of physiology worth understanding. Success in breastfeeding is rooted in the balance of demand and supply—similar, but not identical, to the economic concept. Essentially, the more often a baby nurses, the more milk the mother's body will produce. However, there are limits. A mother who nurses her baby eight times a day will naturally produce more milk than one who nurses only twice, but nursing 12, 15, or even 20 times a day won't necessarily yield more milk than nursing 8-10 times.

The difference lies not in the number of feedings but in the quality of each session. Babies who are on a routine might nurse less frequently, but they take in more calories with each feeding compared to babies who nurse on demand without a set routine. The *PDF* method supports this approach, aiming for full, satisfying feedings that promote steady growth.

To recognize a full feeding, look for these signs:

- enough time spent nursing (10-15 minutes per breast or 20-30 minutes for formula-fed babies),
- the sound of swallowing milk,
- the baby pulling away when satiated,
- a good burp afterward,
- a contented nap.

Babies who only snack, nursing for a few minutes here and there, miss out on these benefits, which can lead to poor nutrition and health risks.

The key to producing enough milk for full feedings is a combination of proper breast stimulation and sufficient time between feedings. Breast stimulation is the vigor of the baby's suckling, driven by hunger. The stronger this drive, the more milk will be produced. Babies who are fed on a regular schedule of every two and a half to three hours tend to have stable digestion and, therefore, demand more milk than babies who snack intermittently throughout the day.

A FEW MORE NURSING FACTS

Breastfeeding success is closely tied to how well a mother cares for her own nutritional needs, particularly her hydration. It's important to eat a balanced diet rich in wholesome fruits, vegetables, grains, protein, and calcium and to drink plenty of fluids. A nursing mother should drink 6-8 ounces of water at each feeding, but avoid drinking too much water, as this can actually harm milk supply. Thirst, concentrated urine, and constipation indicate that more hydration is needed. For the sake of your baby and your own health, stay well hydrated.

The Let-Down Reflex

When a baby begins to nurse, a message is sent to the mother's pituitary gland to release two hormones: prolactin, which is needed for milk production, and oxytocin, which triggers the release of milk. As the baby suckles, the first milk received is the foremilk, which is more diluted and less nutritious. As nursing continues, oxytocin causes the milk glands to contract, releasing the richer hindmilk, which is full of the protein and fat necessary for the baby's growth.

Breastmilk and Baby's Digestion

New mothers may come across various opinions online, such as "Breastmilk is easier to digest than formula, so breastfed babies need to eat more often" or "Breastfed babies cannot sleep through the night because their stomachs empty faster." While there is some truth in the first statement, the second is not accurate. It's not an empty stomach that triggers hunger but the process of digestion and absorption. Efficient digestion, which occurs primarily in the small intestine, allows food molecules to pass into the bloodstream, and as this happens, the blood sugar level drops, signaling to the brain that it's time to eat. Therefore, efficient and full feedings are more important than the type of milk when it comes to satisfying a baby's hunger.

FEEDING AND HYGIENE CONSIDERATIONS

The hands transfer most germs! When it comes to newborn care, keeping your hands clean by washing with soap and water is one of the most important steps of proper hygiene, especially just before feeding your baby. Washing hands with soap and water for a minimum of 20 seconds is the best practice for lifting out and removing germs. We emphasize the use of "soap and water" over hand sanitizer. While very effective, hand sanitizer do not significantly reduce the number of bacteria on the hand, partly because they are not designed to remove dirt like soap and water can.

The commonly cited claim that hand sanitizer can achieve 99% effectiveness is slightly misleading since the claim is based on the product's ability to destroy bacteria on non-porous, hard surfaces and not on hands. When soap and water are unavailable, and you use hand sanitizer, the Center for Disease Control's public website suggests using products that contain at least 60 percent alcohol for maximum hygiene results.

Washing your hands is not just a good practice for Mom and Dad to establish, but it is one to insist on for anyone who will be holding their newborn. With a baby in one's arms, the natural impulse is to touch Baby's face, nose, or chin or hold and examine his little fingers. While touching is part of the human experience, caution dictates hand washing.

PROPER NURSING POSITIONS

The correct positioning of a baby at the breast is essential for successful nursing. A baby should be fully aligned, with the head, chest, stomach, and legs facing the mother's breast. If the baby's head is twisted away, nursing will be inefficient, much like trying to drink with your head turned awkwardly to the side. When the baby is positioned correctly, the tip of the nose will brush against the breast, and the knees will rest on the mother's abdomen.

Once the baby is aligned, the mother should gently stroke the lower lip with her nipple, encouraging the baby to open wide. A wide-open mouth allows the baby to latch onto the areola as well as the nipple, ensuring a proper latch. There are several nursing positions to choose from although we will speak to the three most common. They include the *cradle, side-lying,* or *football hold.*

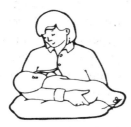

Most commonly used is the *cradle position*. Sitting in a comfortable chair, place your baby's head in the curve of your arm. Placing a pillow under your supporting arm will lessen the stress on your neck and upper back. Remember to keep your baby's entire body properly aligned and facing Mom's breasts.

Mothers recovering from a Cesarean birth will often use the *side-lying position* because of their abdominal sensitivity. The illustration shows Mom in a reclining position with her baby supported by a pillow. The baby and Mom's tummies should be facing each other although not touching. The baby's head should be centered on the breast.

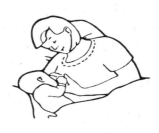

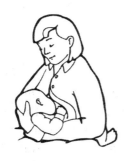

To use the *football hold*, place one hand under Baby's head while lifting and supporting the breast with the other hand. With your fingers above and below the nipple, introduce the baby to the breast by drawing him near. As explained previously, stroke lightly downward on Baby's lower lip until he opens his mouth. When his mouth opens wide, center your nipple and draw him close to you so the tip of his nose is touching your breast.

HOW OFTEN SHOULD I NURSE?

The first rule is always to feed a hungry baby. How often that happens depends on the baby. On average, babies must feed every two to three hours during the first month. The time between feedings is measured from the beginning of one feeding to the beginning of the next, including the time it takes to nurse and the time the baby spends awake and asleep. With this routine, you can expect to feed your baby 8-10 times a day in the early weeks, which aligns with the American Academy of Pediatrics recommendations.[3]

Research shows that babies naturally organize their feeding times into predictable cycles if allowed to do so. A 1941 study found that babies, whether fed on a three-hour schedule, a four-hour schedule, or on demand, tended to prefer a three-hour routine. This inclination toward regularity supports the *PDF* approach, which encourages predictable feeding patterns that help both the baby and the parents.

Time Ranges in a Baby's Day

When discussing feeding times, waketimes, and naps, it's important to remember that these are ranges, not exact numbers. For example, feeding times might fall between two and a half to three hours, and naptimes might range from one to two hours. Some babies will nap for two hours, while others might sleep for just an hour and a half. Both are normal, and it's important not to think of the longer time as better. As long as your baby's activities fall within the normal range, they receive the right amount of time for their needs.

THE THREE MILK PHASES

The first milk produced is a thick, yellowish liquid called *colostrum*. Colostrum is at least five times higher in protein while lower in sugar and fat compared to the more mature breastmilk that has yet to come in. Acting similar to a protein concentrate, colostrum is rich in antibodies that protect the baby from a wide variety of bacterial and viral illnesses. It also encourages the passage of *meconium stool* which is the first stool the baby passes. The meconium stool is greenish black and sticky in texture, comprising everything collected in-utero, including body hair, mucus, bile, and amniotic fluid.

Within 2-4 days, a breastfeeding mother starts to produce a *transition milk*, which can last from 7-14 days. The content of this milk has less protein than colostrum but an increase in fat, lactose, calories, and water-soluble vitamins. The transition milk is followed by regular breastmilk, known as *mature milk.* The mature milk is made up of *foremilk* and *hindmilk,* which contain different quantities of lactose (milk sugars) and fats. The foremilk is released first from the breast and is generally thin in consistency and lower in fat content but higher in lactose, satisfying the baby's thirst and liquid needs.

Hindmilk is released after several minutes of nursing. It is similar in texture to cream and has high-fat levels necessary for weight gain and brain development. Hindmilk also has properties not found in foremilk that help the baby break down and pass waste, establishing healthy elimination patterns.

A Few More Facts

Once the mature milk comes in, nursing periods will average 15 minutes per side. It's not uncommon to experience breast tenderness in the days before mature milk arrives, as the baby's suckling may be more intense while drawing out the thicker colostrum. However, once the milk comes in, the suck-swallow pattern becomes more rhythmic and gentle, easing any discomfort.

The speed at which a baby empties the breast varies. Some babies are quick and efficient, while others take their time. Studies have shown that some babies can empty the breast in as little as 7-10 minutes per side during established lactation. This is not to encourage shorter feeding times, but rather to illustrate a baby's natural ability for efficiency.

Several factors can delay the onset of a strong milk supply, such as a C-section, a stressful birth, or certain medical conditions. However, early, frequent, and effective nursing—especially in the first hours and days after birth—will support the establishment of a good milk supply.

The Very First Nursing Period

The first time a baby is brought to the breast is a moment to treasure. This first nursing period is a special time of bonding, and it's important to simply enjoy the experience. Most babies are alert for the first hour and a half after birth, making it the perfect time to nurse. An initial session of 10-15 minutes per side is often sufficient to stimulate the breasts. Proper positioning is critical to a successful start, helping to prevent soreness and ensuring that both breasts are stimulated at each feeding.

The Sleepy Baby

After the initial period of alertness, babies often become very sleepy, which can make it challenging to ensure they're getting enough to eat. Since newborns need to be fed every 2-3 hours, it's important to rouse a sleepy baby for feeding. Holding the baby skin-to-skin, gently massaging the face, or rubbing the feet can help keep the baby awake long enough to nurse fully. Whispering or sharing your thoughts can also keep the baby engaged during feedings.

Misunderstanding Birth Weight

It's common for parents to be concerned when they hear that their baby has lost weight after birth. This news can be particularly unsettling for mothers who are breastfeeding, leading them to worry about whether they're providing enough nourishment. However, it's important to understand that most babies lose between five and seven percent of their birth weight (sometimes up to 10 percent) within the first few days, and this is entirely normal. This weight loss is mainly due to the loss of excess fluids and the passage of the meconium stool. Knowing the baby's weight at hospital discharge, in addition to the birth weight, can provide reassurance.

Measuring Food Intake

New mothers often wonder if their babies are getting enough to eat. The signs to look for include five to seven wet diapers per day after the first week, three to five or more yellow stools daily during the first month, and steady weight gain. Keeping track of your baby's growth using charts can help you monitor progress and ensure that your little one is thriving.

The First Seven to Ten Days

As noted in Chapter One, the first week or so of nursing is a time of adjustment for both mother and baby. These precious days should be focused on ensuring full feedings rather than worrying about strict schedules. Many mothers find that after a week of consistent, full feedings, their babies naturally settle into a 2½ to 3-hour routine. The length of nursing sessions may vary, with some newborns nursing faster and others taking a bit longer.

How Long Is a Nursing Period?

Some mothers nurse their babies for 15-20 minutes on one side, burp them, and then offer the second side for an additional 15-20 minutes. Other mothers employ a 10-10-5-5 method. They alternate sides, offer each breast for 10 minutes (burping the baby between sides), and then offer each breast for five additional minutes. This second method is helpful if Mom has a sleepy baby, as the disruption prompts the baby to wakefulness and assures that both breasts are stimulated equally. During these early days, if baby desires to nurse longer, Mom can let him do so or consider using a pacifier. If she feels her baby has a need for non-nutritive sucking, a pacifier can nicely meet this need without compromising the routine or making Mom feel like she is becoming a pacifier.

UNDERSTANDING GROWTH SPURTS

Sometimes, even with regular full feedings, a baby will seem hungrier than usual. This often happens during a growth spurt, a period when the baby's body needs extra calories to support rapid development. Growth spurts, also referred to as *leaps*, tend to occur at predictable times, such as around ten days, three weeks, six weeks, three months, and six months. During these times, the baby may need to feed more frequently, and parents may notice increased fussiness or shorter naps A three hour feeding routine might become a two or two and a-half hour routine for two or three days.

Growth spurts can be challenging for new mothers, lasting anywhere from one to four days. However, once the growth spurt is over, normal feeding and sleeping patterns typically resume, although Baby may nap longer for a few days.

For a new mom, the challenge is recognizing the onset of that first growth spurt. Other than a pre-set alarm notice, there is usually no warning before it happens. Just as the feed-wake-sleep routine is finally falling into place, one day she is hit by a growth-spurt snowball! Mom will notice an all-of-a-sudden increase in hunger signs, along with excessive fussiness and waking about 40-50 minutes early from his nap with a ravenous appetite. Mom feeds, puts Baby back down for a nap and the whole thing repeats itself in 2 hours or less.

How will a Mom know when the growth spurt is over? Normal feeding cycles will resume, and the next day, Baby will nap longer than normal. That is because growth spurts are fatiguing for babies as much as they are for mothers.

BOTTLE FEEDING WITH FORMULA

For some mothers, formula feeding is the best or only option, and this choice should be respected. Feeding a baby with formula does not reflect negatively on a mother's care or ability, just as breastfeeding does not automatically make one a good mother. The important thing is the love and attention with which the baby is fed. Parents should take the time to cuddle during bottle feedings, which provides not only nourishment but also the emotional connection the baby needs.

During the first half of the twentieth century, when bottle feeding was in vogue, selections were limited, but today, that is not the case. Store shelves are filled with options, from standard glass and plastic bottles to those with disposable bags, handles and animal shapes. All come in a wide range of colors and prints, although this is more for the mother's amusement than the baby's.

The variety of nipple types ranges from a nipple most like Mom to an orthodontic nipple, a juice nipple, and even one for cereal (which we do not recommend). The most important feature is the right-sized hole. A nipple hole that is too large forces Baby to drink too fast, which often leads to excessive spitting up and projectile vomiting. A hole that is too small creates a hungry and discontented baby. To test the nipple, turn the bottle upside down. There should be a slow drip of formula. If the formula flows freely, the hole is too big.

One advantage to bottle feeding is that it allows others to participate. Feeding the baby can be just as special for Dad as it is for Mom. Fathers should not be denied this opportunity to nurture their babies. The same holds true for age-appropriate siblings and grandparents. It is a family affair, and everyone benefits.[4]

FORMULA

Formula is designed to approximate the nutritional qualities of breast-milk and comes in various types, including milk-based, soy-based, and *hypoallergenic* options. It's important to consult with a pediatrician to determine the best formula for your baby. Formula is available in powder, liquid concentrate, and ready-to-feed forms, each with its own advantages and considerations.

Be aware that cow's milk and baby formula are not the same. Cow's milk is not suitable for children under a year of age. The best source of information about which formula is best for your baby is your pediatrician or family practitioner. Do not be shy about asking questions.

The Food and Drug Administration (FDA) oversees the manufacturing of infant formulas, ensuring the end product complies with nutritional requirements. Baby formula is sold in three different forms:

- Powder: the least expensive form, mixed with water.

- Liquid concentrate: mixed with an equal amount of water.(Easier to work with than powder.)

- Ready-to-feed: expensive but does not require mixing.

How much formula should your baby consume? The AAP provides a handy guide that should be followed. It states babies should receive 2½ ounces of formula for each pound of body weight. For example, if your baby weighs 13 pounds, then he should be receiving approximately 32 ounces of formula in a 24-hour period. Once a baby is sleeping through the night (at least 8 hours), then that would work out to 6-8 ounces every 3-4 hours during the day, but should not exceed the daily portion of 32 ounces, unless otherwise directed by your baby's pediatrician.

Bottle Feeding Positions to Avoid

Avoid bottle feeding a baby while he is lying completely flat. (This also applies to moms tempted to nurse in a lying-down position.) Taking liquids while lying down may allow fluid to enter the middle ear, leading to ear infections. Putting a baby to bed with a bottle is also a no-no, not only because of ear infections but also to prevent tooth decay. When a baby falls asleep with a bottle in his mouth, the sugar in the formula coats the teeth, resulting in tooth decay even when baby teeth are developing.

Formula is designed to approximate the nutritional qualities of breastmilk and comes in various types, including milk-based, soy-based, and hypoallergenic options. It's essential to consult with a pediatrician to determine the best formula for your baby. Formula is available in powder, liquid concentrate, and ready-to-feed forms, each with its own advantages and considerations.

BURPING YOUR BABY

Feeding and burping a baby are inseparably linked because babies will always swallow some air as they feed, and, if the air is not discharged, it will lead to discomfort. Inside Baby's tummy, the swallowed air exists in the form of tiny bubbles that cannot escape or be released without help. Patting a baby's back in conjunction with applying slight pressure to his tummy forces the smaller bubbles to collect, forming one larger bubble that the baby is able to burp up.

There are four common positions for burping a baby. Find the one that is most effective for you and your baby, while staying mindful that the process of burping may occur one, two, or three times during a feeding, depending on the baby and the efficiency of his feeding. Bottle-fed newborns will need to be burped after every 1-2 ounces, and breastfed babies when changing sides.

1. <u>Sitting Lap Position</u>: Place the palm of your hand over Baby's stomach. Now hook your thumb around the side of your baby, wrapping

the rest of your fingers around the chest area. Note how the baby is securely resting upright on Mom's lap with one of her hands supporting and holding his chest. Lean your baby slightly and begin patting.

2. <u>Tummy-over-Lap Position</u>: In a sitting position, place your baby's legs between your legs and drape the baby over your thigh. While supporting the baby's head in your hands, bring your knees together for further support and pat Baby's back firmly.

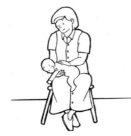

3. <u>The Shoulder Position</u>: With Baby's chest resting on a cloth diaper high on Mom's shoulder and his tummy resting on the front of her shoulder, begin patting Baby's back firmly.

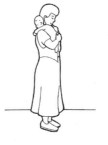

4. <u>The Cradle Position</u>: Mom cradles the baby in her arm with his bottom in her hands and his head resting at Mom's elbow. One of the

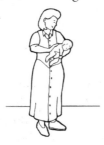

baby's arms and one leg are to be wrapped around her arm, making sure the baby is facing away from her. This position allows her other hand to be free to pat the baby's back.

Note: If a baby does not burp after a few minutes, Mom should consider changing the baby's burping position and try again before she continues the feeding. Without a doubt, Mom will want to keep her clothing clean, so keeping a cloth diaper handy when burping will have its rewards.

Burping Challenges

During the first week of life, when a baby tends to be more sleepy, it is sometimes difficult to get a baby to burp. If, after trying for 5 minutes, the baby is more interested in sleeping than burping, place her in the infant seat rather than her crib. Gravity is a wonderful thing, helping to keep the milk down and eventually causing the air bubbles to dissipate. After each feeding—with the exceptions of the late-evening feeding and middle-of-the-night feeding—placing the newborn in an infant seat for 10-15 minutes helps prevent the milk from refluxing up into the esophagus. Elevating the head of your newborn's crib by an inch or two can also be helpful, especially if your little one has a mild case of reflux. Simply place a book or board under each leg at the head of the crib.

Spitting Up and Projectile Vomiting

Spitting up is a common occurrence with infants. It usually occurs during the burping process when the "bubble" is released and some of the ingested milk also comes up with the burp. It can also happen because of unnecessary motion, such as when Grandpa bounces Baby on his knee or big sister tries to soothe Baby by excessive swaying in a rocking motion. When spitting up occurs because of motion, it usually signals that a baby has eaten more food than the stomach can process at one time. As the stomach pressure builds, spitting up is the mechanism to release the excess. There is no reason to be alarmed over this, but Mom should monitor how often this is happening and, if she needs to, reduce the number of ounces her baby receives.

A more alarming form of spitting up is called "projectile vomiting," which is much greater in volume and very forceful, traveling 4-6 feet across a room. Projectile vomiting is not a particular diagnosis or condition but a comparative term to the much less intense dribbling type of spitting up. Although any baby can have a bout or two of projectile vomiting, routine episodes indicate a more serious problem. Projectile vomiting can be a sign of gastroesophageal reflux, (see Appnedix B).

It can also indicate an intestinal infection. The baby who routinely vomits his meals will not receive enough calories for adequate growth and can quickly become dehydrated. Establishing a correct diagnosis and treatment is very important. Do not be shy regarding contacting your health care provider, when in doubt or have questions, especially healthy related questions.

Hiccups

Even with the best burping techniques, there will be times when an air bubble becomes trapped in a baby's tummy or intestines, resulting in one of two outcomes: hiccups or passing gas. Unfortunately, with the latter sensation, most babies react by tightening their bottoms and resisting the normal expulsion of passing gas, making themselves very uncomfortable. To alleviate your baby's discomfort, place him in a knee-chest position or place his back next to your chest, then pull his knees up to his chest.

Every baby goes through a bout or two of hiccups, and some experience them daily, even in the womb. After birth, hiccups in babies are quite normal and more troublesome to the parents than the baby. Hiccups can range from 5-30 minutes in length, and while no scientific certainty can be attributed to the cause, most evidence points to feeding. If you notice your newborn is hiccupping after each feeding, try offering a little less formula or breastmilk while feeding slightly more often and see if that makes a difference. Another idea is to treat the hiccups like a burp. Using one of the upright burping positions, gently pat your baby on his back; the release of some remaining trapped air could relieve the problem.

TO THE POINT

In these moments of feeding, whether from breast or bottle, a mother's love shines brightest, nurturing not only the body but also the heart and soul of her little one. The simple acts of care and attention are the building blocks of a strong and healthy start in life, creating a bond that will grow ever stronger with time.

Chapter Seven

Responding To Your Baby's Cry

W hen your baby's cry slices through the stillness of your home, it is as if the very air trembles with the weight of that sound. It resonates not just within the walls but within your heart, a primal call that seems to echo across the universe. Yet, nestled within that cry is a hidden message—a plea for help, comfort, or perhaps something less urgent but no less critical. The true challenge for every parent lies in unraveling the mystery of that cry, in deciphering the subtle nuances that reveal its true meaning.

Beyond the hunger that might drive your baby to tears, there exists a multitude of reasons—a symphony of needs that can range from the simple discomfort of tiredness or illness to the restless stirring of boredom, frustration, or a longing for the familiar embrace of routine. At times, a baby cries with no apparent cause, perhaps merely the weariness of a day too full or too empty.

No parent welcomes this sound, especially when stepping into the tender role of caretaker for the first time. A baby's cry stirs within you a profound uncertainty unlike anything you have ever known. It is a force that shakes you to your core, making you question if something vital has been overlooked or if an invisible mistake has been made. It breeds moments of anxious self-doubt, leaving you to wonder, If only I knew what to do!

Yet, take solace, for even the American Academy of Pediatrics acknowledges that crying is an intrinsic part of a baby's daily existence. They offer reassurance in their vast tome of infant care: "All babies cry, often without any discernible reason. Newborns typically cry for a total of 1 to 4 hours a day. No mother can console her child whenever he cries, so do not burden yourself with the expectation of performing miracles. Pay close attention to your baby's different cries, and soon you will discern when he needs to be held, comforted, or cared for and when he might simply need to be left alone."[1]

Think of crying not as a judgment upon your parenting but as a language—a way for your baby to communicate the depths of their need. As a mother and father, your journey is to become fluent in this language and respond with tenderness and understanding. The ability to interpret your baby's cries will instill confidence within you as a parent and weave a stronger bond between you and your child, a bond that grows with each cry answered, with each need met. But how does one unlock the secrets of these cries?

In those early months, crying becomes the voice of need and discomfort, yet these are different. Each requires its delicate response, a dance of intuition and care that only you can learn to master.

Cry of Discomfort

A cry of discomfort often arises from immediate, physical unease. This cry might emerge from something as simple as being in an uncomfortable position or feeling too hot or cold. For example, a baby might cry in discomfort when a diaper is too tight, when lying in an awkward position, or when needing a burp. The cry is not so much about a deeper need but rather about alleviating an immediate, often surface-level irritation.

Cry of Need

In contrast, the cry for need carries a weightier significance. While both cries demand attention, the cry of discomfort often seeks immediate, yet simple, relief, whereas the cry for need calls for something more profound. This response addresses a variety of fundamental needs. The cry of hunger differs from the cry of sickness, just as sleepiness is distinct from the cry that asks for a cuddle. There are cries of distress and cries of demand, and they vary in intensity. Sometimes, it's a soft whimper; other times, it's a vigorous protest. Understanding the difference between these cries allows a parent to offer the appropriate comfort or intervention.

.THE INEVITABLE CONFLICT

To suppress or diminish your baby's tears by offering more food is to attempt to quiet the storm without addressing the gathering clouds. Such a strategy, far from easing the turmoil, can deepen both your baby's distress and your own. In the vast, often contradictory world of parenting advice, two extremes beckon like treacherous sirens: those who urge you to let your baby "cry it out" and those who demand that you silence every cry. Both paths lead you astray, pulling you away from the anchoring wisdom of your own instincts, binding you instead to the rigid chains of ideology.

The first extreme, rooted in the Behaviorist movement of the early 20th century, viewed the well-scheduled child as the pinnacle of parental success, even if that meant ignoring the plaintive wails of genuine hunger or need. This was a time when the child's cries were seen not as a call for care but as a battle to be won through discipline and order.

In contrast, the Attachment Parenting philosophy of the late 20th century swung to the opposite pole, preaching that all crying must be stifled, driven by the misguided belief that a baby's tears are echoes of anxiety rooted in birth trauma. Here, the cry was not a signal to be understood but a symptom to be eradicated.

Yet, as with most things in life, the truth lies not in these extremes but somewhere in the delicate balance between them. Research has shown that infants allowed to cry during the normal rhythms of infancy grow into robust, resourceful individuals—children who, when confronted with challenges, find within themselves the strength and ingenuity to overcome them, secure in the knowledge that their parents are there, neither anxious nor afraid.[2]

On the other hand, babies whose cries are constantly hushed may lose the drive to solve problems on their own, learning instead to wait passively for rescue. This hints at a deeper truth: infants begin to understand the connection between their actions and the world's responses when crying is managed with sensitivity rather than suppressed.

A Measure of Comfort

Throughout the day, you'll naturally hold your baby often—whether during feedings, while rocking them gently in your arms, or simply in those quiet moments of cuddling. This close contact is essential, a balm that provides comfort and reassurance, wrapping your little one in the warmth of your love. Whether in joy or in fussiness, your baby revels in the attention. Who wouldn't? Yet, it is important to remember that it's easy to overdo this attention, especially when your baby is feeling fussy.

As parents, our instinct is to offer comfort when comfort is needed, but the true wisdom lies in discerning what kind of comfort is truly required. A wet diaper is best soothed by a fresh one. A hungry baby finds solace in a feeding. A startled baby finds peace in the embrace of loving arms, and a tired baby needs the gentle surrender of sleep. These associations form the bedrock of more intricate skills, such as self-soothing and problem-solving.

Comfort can take many forms—rocking, a soft lullaby, a stroll in the fresh air, or the soothing notes of music nearby. This comfort can come from many sources as well, not just from you, but from Dad, older siblings, Grandma, and Grandpa, each offering their unique touch of love.

A mother's wisdom lies in recognizing that a baby responds to different forms of comfort at different times. If you rely solely on one source, such as nursing, you may not be truly comforting your baby but merely quieting their cry by triggering the sucking reflex. When nursing becomes the only form of comfort, other real needs may remain unfulfilled, leaving your baby's deeper needs unmet.

By attempting to silence every cry, parents may inadvertently rob their little one of the opportunity to develop these essential patterns of learning, denying them the chance to discover that their actions, their very voice, have power and meaning in this world. We find the true art of comforting our children in the variety and thoughtfulness of our responses.

UNDERSTANDING YOUR BABY'S CRY

The secret to truly understanding and responding to a baby's cry lies in hearing the cry and interpreting the world surrounding it. It is in the art of reading the context, the unspoken language that accompanies those tears. When a baby cries, the first question a parent should ask is not simply Why is my baby crying? But rather, "What has shifted in my baby's world that needs attention? "What variable in the baby's life right now needs assessment?" Without this delicate assessment, parents may be overwhelmed, misreading the signals and offering responses totally disconnected from the baby's real needs.

In the tender span of the first five months, there are six distinct moments when crying emerges—three of these are cries that fall into the realm of the abnormal, signaling that something is amiss and demands immediate action. The other three are cries of a different nature, natural expressions that, while still important signals, call for a more measured, thoughtful response.

Let us now delve into each of these cries, exploring their meanings and the wisdom required to respond to them with the care and understanding that nurtures both the child and the bond you share.

Abnormal Sounding Cries

While some crying is normal, certain sounding cries should alert you to potential issues. A high-pitched, piercing cry might indicate pain or injury and should be brought to your pediatrician's attention. A sudden change in your baby's crying pattern, such as increased frequency or a weaker cry, could be a sign of illness and should be discussed with a healthcare professional.

Abnormal Cry Periods

Crying during feedings, immediately after feedings, and in the middle of a sound nap are all abnormal and should be investigated promptly.

Crying During Feeding: This is not what one would expect in the gentle rhythm of a feeding. Has your baby become frustrated or overwhelmed? Perhaps the milk flows too quickly, like a rushing river, or too slowly, like a trickling stream. There are many possible reasons behind this distress—improper latching or a hesitant release of milk among them. Each possibility a clue, each cry a question waiting to be answered.

Crying Immediately After Feeding: If your baby's cries begin within thirty minutes of a feeding and the sound is more a cry of pain than of drowsy contentment, there may be hidden discomfort. Trapped gas, that stubborn and unseen foe, or perhaps something in the mother's diet, especially dairy or spicy foods, might be the culprits causing digestive unrest in your little one. Keeping a food diary, like a detective's notebook, may help uncover the source of this discomfort. And for mothers who breastfeed, consider the quality of your milk—if doubts arise, do not hesitate to seek the wisdom of your pediatrician.

Crying in the Middle of a Sound Nap: When a baby is roused from the depths of a peaceful sleep with a piercing cry, it is as if some unseen force has disturbed their dreams. Perhaps it is trapped gas, a sudden shift in their routine, or even a subtle decrease in milk supply that has awakened them so abruptly. In these moments, feeding may indeed soothe their distress, but it is equally important to look beyond the surface and investigate the root cause of this interruption in their slumber.

Normal Cry Periods

Other types of crying, such as just before feeding, during the late-afternoon or early-evening period, and when being put down for a nap or bedtime, fall into the normal category and should be expected.

Crying Just Before Feeding: This is usually brief, as mealtime is near. If your baby consistently shows signs of hunger before the scheduled feeding, it's worth investigating why rather than letting them cry it out.

Crying During the Late-Afternoon/Early-Evening Period: Many babies have a "fussy time" during this period. If your baby becomes exceptionally fussy and is not comforted by usual methods, consider whether they might be hungry or if there is something in your diet that could be affecting them.

Crying When Going Down for a Nap: When your baby is laid down for a nap, the length of their crying is a melody composed by the child, though carefully watched over by the parent. For some little ones, crying becomes a kind of art, an expressive symphony that fills the room, even when they are surrounded by love, tenderness, and the most devoted care.

More About Crying

There are babies who, despite every effort to comfort them, seem to be born with a greater inclination to cry, particularly when it is time to surrender to sleep. This does not signify that their fundamental needs are unmet; rather, it speaks to a certain temperament, a disposition to cry that we, as parents, might wish were otherwise. Yet, it is a part of who they are, a characteristic as innate as the color of their eyes or the sound of their laughter, a reminder that each child carries within them their own unique way of expressing to the world around them. The American Academy of Pediatrics (AAP) recognizes this fact: "Many babies cannot fall asleep without crying and will go to sleep more quickly if left to cry for a while. The crying should not last long if the child is truly tired."[3]

It is not unusual for a sleeping baby to occasionally whimper or cry softly in the middle of a nap. Again, the words of the AAP are helpful in understanding what might be going on: "Sometimes you may think your baby is waking up when he is actually going through a phase of very light slumber. He could be startled, squirming, fussing, or even crying—and still be asleep. Or he may be awake but on the verge of drifting off again if left alone. Do not make the mistake of trying to immediately intervene during these moments; you will only awaken him further and delay him from going back to sleep. Instead, if you let him fuss and even cry for a few minutes, he will learn to get himself to sleep without relying on you."[4]

The AAP goes on to say that "some babies actually need to let off energy by crying in order to settle into sleep or rouse themselves out of it. As much as fifteen to twenty minutes of fussing will not do your child any harm. Just be sure he is not crying out of hunger or pain, or because his diaper is wet."[5]

In the pursuit of instilling good sleep habits, a measure of temporary crying is a small price to pay compared to the far-reaching consequences of poor or underdeveloped nighttime sleep patterns. The gentle art of sleep training, though it may bring some tears in the beginning, offers lasting benefits that echo through the early months and beyond. It diminishes the frequency of crying as the year progresses, not to mention the struggles of sleepless nights.

A well-rested baby is a contented feeder, one who drifts off to sleep with ease when laid down for a nap or bedtime. You can walk away, confident that your child will slip into slumber and awaken with a smile, refreshed and peaceful. Another blessing of this approach is its universality—you can lay your baby down in any home, and the same serene ritual will unfold, free from the disruptions that unfamiliar surroundings might bring.

Some babies cry for five minutes before they surrender to sleep's embrace, while others may vary their cries from a brief five minutes to a more drawn-out, intermittent fifteen minutes. If your baby's crying stretches beyond fifteen minutes, it is wise to check on them. A gentle pat on the back, perhaps a moment of holding, and then back to bed they go.

Remember, your goal is not to silence your baby's cries but to teach them the sacred skill of sleep. This might be the only time in their day when the best response is no response at all, allowing them to discover the quiet power of settling themselves into sleep.

TO THE POINT

As you become more attuned to your baby's cries, you'll start to recognize patterns. Some babies have a naptime cry that follows a predictable pattern—a gentle whimper that builds to a wail, then subsides as sleep takes over. Others might cry in short bursts, stopping and starting before falling asleep. Over time, you'll learn what is normal for your baby. While abnormal cries should be addressed immediately, other cries can be approached with the following steps:

Consider Your Baby's Routine. Is it feeding time, the end of waketime, or the beginning of naptime, or is he waking in the middle of a nap? Discerning where your little one is in his routine will help you determine the cause and best respond accordingly.

Listen for the Type of Cry: Pay attention to the tone and pattern of the cry. Sometimes, the crying will stop as quickly as it started. By listening carefully, you not only decide on the best response but also learn the habits of your baby's cry.

Take Action: Sometimes, the best action is no action at all. If your baby is fed, clean, and ready for sleep, they may need to learn how to fall asleep on their own. However, if the crying persists, it may be necessary to check on them. If your baby is stuck in a corner of the crib, gently move them and offer a comforting pat before leaving the room.

There will be times when holding and comforting your baby is the right response, even if it's just to offer reassurance. The key is to assess each situation and respond in a way that meets your baby's needs without creating unnecessary dependencies. A delicate balance for sure.

Chapter Eight

Topic Pool For New Parents

When a couple discovers they are expecting, at first, very little seems to shift in their daily lives. The familiar rhythm of their routines—work, home, and all the duties in between—continues as it always has. Mom will make some gradual adjustments as the baby grows within, but overall, life on the pre-birth side of things is much easier than after delivery. Then comes Baby!

This is when the world shifts, and the delicate balance tilts in ways that no couple can fully anticipate. Though the chances are good that the pregnancy and birth will be smooth, the truth is that when a baby enters the home, nothing goes exactly as Mom and Dad envisioned. Here is where expectations and reality often collide.

It's a sweet illusion to believe things will be different for them than for the struggling couple down the street. Most women possess a quiet confidence that their pregnancy will be different, their ability to manage a newborn will be without challenge, their home life will quickly return to normal, and their baby will respond with sweet smiles and contented coos to every motherly gesture of love and care.

While we have no desire to dampen anyone's enthusiasm or hopeful expectations, we offer this caution to help you: the more you leave room in your thinking that babyhood comes with a few unplanned disruptions, the better you will be able to adjust when the unexpected invades your baby's day. Parents who assume they can plan and control every moment without some intrusive disruption will feel disappointed. By accepting the reality that they cannot, in a God-like fashion, control all outcomes of their baby's life, they are accepting the finite of humanity. Over time, they will learn to embrace the unknown, to dance with the unexpected, and to find joy even in the surprises that parenthood brings.

To help ease the transitions that a baby introduces, we will now explore a series of considerations that may help parents prepare. Some ideas may feel familiar, others will be new, but all are offered in the spirit of preparing hearts and minds for the beautiful chaos that is to come.

ACHIEVEMENT LEVELS

All humans are uniquely different, yet we share developmental similarities that serve as a basis for achievement levels. A basic routine enhances learning because order and predictability are natural allies of the learning process. Keeping in mind the ripple-effect principle spoken of in Chapter Two, good routines encourage healthy sleep, and good sleepers experience optimal alertness during waketimes. That facilitates how they interact with their environment. As a result, these children are self-assured and happy, less demanding and more pleasant, secure and healthy. They have longer attention spans, possess self-control and focusing skills, and, as a result, become faster learners.

There is a beautiful diversity within infant development, which means infants may achieve new levels at slightly different ages. If your baby seems to be progressing at a different pace than your neighbor's baby, there's no need to worry. One baby might cut a tooth at four months, while another might do so at six months. This is not a problem, just a natural difference, reflected in the range of norms you will see in baby books (including this one).

If, however, your baby does not achieve a skill within the norm tables of expectations, that could signal a muscular or neurologic problem. For example, pediatricians are concerned when a full-term two-month-old cannot lift his head while lying on his tummy. They are also concerned if a full-term three-month-old is crossing his legs when lifted under his arms or if his neck lacks muscle control to support his head when picked up from a back-lying position. Understanding the various developmental markers of growth can help parents make a general assessment of their baby's progress. If you sense your baby is lagging behind developmentally, consult your healthcare provider. The term developmental delay is applied to infants who are not growing according to established norms.

Premature infants, who make up about 12 percent of U.S. babies, have a different set of norms and may lag behind full-term infants in achievement levels up through the first two years. However, it's important to remember that they usually catch up with full-term babies in every category of development by age two, bringing hope and optimism to their parents.

BABY EQUIPMENT
It is easy to walk into a baby superstore and get caught up with the new, the pretty, and the fancy. Baby equipment and accessories are marketed to parents' likes and preferences. In truth, your baby doesn't care about fashion. It is simply not on their radar, so do not worry if your budget does not support new or pretty. In truth, except for car seat and the crib, most baby equipment is optional. Many items, including the high chair, stroller, changing table, and crib, can be borrowed from a relative or friend or found at a garage sale.

Baby Monitor
Audio baby monitors first came on the scene in the 1960s. Today's generation of monitors now includes video capability. Parents can hear and see what is happening in the baby's room. The price tags range from $30 for a simple monitor without video to $400 if you are looking for high-definition color and night vision.

Some kind of monitor is worth the investment because it allows you to monitor your baby from a distance. This provides Mom and Dad the freedom to move around the house while Baby is in his crib, playpen, or alone in his room. A potential downside is that hearing every little sigh, noise, whimper, or stirring of your baby may be cute initially but can become wearying. And in the still of the night, monitors magnify every sound, leaving parents in exhaustion by morning. The last thing a baby needs in the morning is a cranky parent, so consider turning the sound control down at night. Be aware that baby monitors are not medical devices and are not intended or able to prevent SIDS.

Car Seat

The car seat is an item that will be around for a while, so think long-term when making this investment. Some car seats are very stylish and work fine with an infant but may not be practical for a growing toddler. Do some comparison shopping to avoid having to purchase a second car seat.

For first-time parents, it's essential to understand the additional attention to be paid to protect your baby while traveling in his car seat. To prevent your baby's head from rolling side to side and potentially causing damage to his neck muscles, consider moving a cloth diaper or receiving a blanket to support each side of the baby's head. Or you can purchase special inserts made for car seats. Whatever you choose, be sure the items do not block your baby's breathing.

With precious cargo on board, you will drive cautiously and defensively, being mindful that sudden stops impact babies most of all because they lack neck-muscle strength. Infants and toddlers should ride in a rear-facing seat until they reach the weight or height designated for their car safety seat manufacturer. Most seats allow children to ride rear-facing for at least two years.

However, different countries have different rules, so please check your local government authority to see current safety requirements. For example, in Australia, children need to stay rear-facing until about 12 months and in a car seat until around seven years of age.

Crib

Cribs and cradles are not products of the Industrial Revolution but furniture that has been around for thousands of years. Ancient Mediterranean societies from Greece, Rome, and Israel used cribs for their babies. The cradle, an infant crib with rocking motion, gained popularity in the Middle Ages and became a status symbol of wealth. Mothers in primitive settings hung cribs from the ceiling of their huts, where they could gently rock their babies as they passed by. The crib is the most essential piece of baby furniture you will own. Give thought to the one you will buy or borrow since your child will spend nearly half the first 18 months of his life in it.

A firm, good-quality mattress should fit snugly against all four sides of the crib. A snug fit prevents the baby from getting any body parts stuck between the bed and the crib. The guardrail should be at least 26 inches/65 cm above the top of the mattress to discourage any attempt to climb out when the baby is older.

The spaces between the crib slats should be at most 2 and 3/8 inches/6 cm apart. Avoid placing the crib near drafty windows, heaters, or air ducts. A steady blast of hot air can dry out your baby's nose and throat, leading to respiratory problems. The American Academy of Pediatrics (AAP) does not recommend placing a baby to sleep on a soft surface such as a water bed, pillow, or soft mattress.

Infant Seat

This is not a car seat. An infant seat is a lightweight, portable seat made especially for infants. You can use it from day one and find it more valuable than any other equipment in the early weeks and months. Infant seats often come with chair straps for safety's sake, making them suitable for feeding your baby solids when the time comes. While the highchair will be used most of the time, the infant seat is handy, especially when visiting friends or at a restaurant..

Infant Swings

Some infant swings play music while they rock, and others offer various reclining options and multiple speeds. Babies going through fussy times tend to soothe more quickly in a swing set at a fast pace, whereas a slower speed is conducive to relaxed, non-fussy times. The reclining swing also works well after feeding to help relieve pressure in Baby's full tummy.

The AAP recommends not using the swing until your baby can sit up on his own, usually by 7-8 months of age. Most grandmothers, however, will tell you that once your baby has good head and upper-back control, the swing can be introduced in the reclining position, as long as the baby is propped well and firmly secured so he cannot move or slip out of the swing. A swing should not be used for long periods, no more than 15-20 minutes twice a day, and never outside Mom or Dad's visual range.

Whether you purchase a new swing or borrow one from a friend, make sure it is assembled well, has a broad base, and has a low center of gravity. While tipping over is rare, it can happen if the swing is not centered correctly and your baby leans too far over in one direction. Use the lap and shoulder belts faithfully—they are there to protect your baby!

BATHING YOUR BABY

There are two types of baths: the sponge bath, recommended until the umbilical cord falls off and the belly button area is healed, around (5-15 days) and the full bath. A sponge bath is like a regular bath, except you do not submerge a baby in water.

Whether in a sponge or a full bath, newborns do not need a bath every day. It is recommended that they have no more than three per week for the first month. There are two reasons for this recommendation. First, newborns do not sweat or have a long enough waketime to get dirty, and second, over-bathing can dry out a baby's delicate skin.

While some countries differ on the timing of Baby's first full bath (based on umbilical cord concerns), the American Academy of Pediatrics recommends sponge baths until the cord falls off. Once that happens, the baby is ready for a full bath in the kitchen sink (easier on the parent's back) or plastic tub lined with a clean towel. Two or three inches / 5-8 cm of water is all that is needed in the basin, and be sure the water temperature is warm to your wrist but not hot. There are some cautions to consider when it comes to soap. Use it sparingly because it can dry out a baby's skin, rinse your baby frequently to remove any soap residue, and use only mild, neutral-pH soaps without additives.

Bathing a baby starts with the head and face region and then the extremities. Use a soft washcloth around your baby's face and head, especially the area over the baby's fontanelles (soft spot on the head.) Apply a slow gentle motion. Never scrub a baby's skin and never leave a baby unattended, even after he is capable of sitting up by himself. The potential danger is too great a risk, even for a minute. These safety measures are designed to give you peace of mind and ensure your baby's well-being..

BLANKET TIME
It may be hard to imagine that learning could be taking place when a five-month-old baby is stretched out on his blanket, playing with a colorful toy or teething ring, yet it is true; blanket time facilitates early learning by allowing a baby to concentrate and serves as a practical mobile boundary. You can begin blanket time with your baby as soon as he can hold his head up and manipulate an object in his hands, as early as four months. Start with 5-10 minutes once a day and stretch the time to a level contentedly accepted by your baby. The beauty of a blanket is its mobility. You can place it anywhere in the house, convenient for Mom and Dad. Grandparents will also find it helpful when the baby is over for a visit.

BONDING WITH YOUR BABY
The term "bonding" evolved from a controversial theory in the 1980s relating to mothers and their babies into common usage today to describe two people emotionally connecting. The original theory postulated that a sensitive period exists for the mother soon after birth when she must make eye-to-eye and skin-to-skin contact with her baby for a long-term maternal connection to take place truly.

Most couples assume this bonding is for the baby's benefit, but the original theory focuses on the mom, suggesting that if she fails to make an immediate connection right after birth, she is more likely to reject her baby passively by withholding love and nurturing. Before worrying about the poor mom who does not have the chance to hold her baby immediately after delivery, be aware that research has not substantiated the cause-and-effect relationship this theory speaks of. Although some animals show instinctive tendencies, speculating that rational beings respond similarly is scientifically unacceptable. Anthropology, the study of humankind, is very different from zoology, the study of animals.[1]

The shortsightedness of the bonding theory, however, should not take away from the beautiful moment right after birth when Mom, Dad and Baby meet for the first time. It's a moment filled with joy, touch, tears, photos, and soft words of affection. If Mom and Baby are temporarily separated at birth, her love as a mother will not diminish, nor will her child move through life permanently impaired because of a bonding deficit created in the first few hours or even days after birth.[2]

CESAREAN BIRTH

This method of delivery, commonly referred to as a C-section, is accomplished through an incision in the abdominal wall and uterus. The decision to perform a C-section is made either before your due date because of a known condition or unexpected complication or during labor because of an unforeseen complication. In either case, competent doctors have your best interests in mind.

Often, a first-time mom goes into labor before having a C-section, which means her body must endure two major events, and so must the Baby. Infants born by emergency C-sections tend to experience a bit more sluggishness or fussiness for the first few weeks. They may be cranky because of medications Mom must take post-op, but typically, everything settles down by the third week. C-section babies experience no delays in sleeping through the night in the *PPD* population, although they tend to be closer to the 8-10 week mark.

Because a Cesarean birth is a major surgery, give yourself time to heal when you get home with the Baby. When he naps, make sure you nap, too. Household chores can wait. However, some things do not change with a Cesarean birth. Loving and nurturing your Baby is one of them.

More C-sections are performed today because medical science has developed more excellent technology for protecting babies, but also because there are more lawsuits against obstetricians and gynecologists, forcing them to exercise conservative, lower-risk treatment. Having a C-section is a medical decision that does not reflects on a woman's motherhood. The goal of a C-section is a healthy outcome.

CRADLE CAP

Adults shed skin cells frequently without noticing. With babies, the new skin cells grow rapidly and often faster than the old cells can fall off, leaving the old cells stuck to the new ones. It appears as a white, scaly, or patchy rash when this happens. It tends to occur most often on a baby's head, ears, and forehead, and it has acquired the name cradle cap. It is not dangerous or contagious and bothers Mom and Dad more than Baby. Your healthcare provider will probably recommend a cream, along with the advice to monitor it, but not to worry about it.

CRIB DEATH (SIDS)

The unexpected death of a healthy baby is referred to as Sudden Infant Death Syndrome (SIDS) or crib death. It is responsible for about 7,000 reported deaths a year worldwide, and it is neither predictable nor preventable from what we currently know. There are more male victims, especially among those who are born prematurely, and it occurs more often among babies of certain ethnic groups, young single mothers, and homes with at least one smoker. A child can be a victim of SIDS at any time during the first year, but the highest percentage occurs between months two and four. More babies die of SIDS during the winter months and in colder climates.

The research strongly suggests that putting a baby on his back for sleep rather than on his tummy reduces the risk of SIDS.[3] What is not conclusive is whether sleeping on his back is the primary or secondary factor in reducing risk. Is the risk removed because the child sleeps on his back, which keeps his mouth and nose from directly laying on soft surfaces and gas-trapping objects (mattresses, pillows, crib liners)? Could those items be the actual sources of SIDS or is the problem connected to the biomechanics of tummy sleeping?

More research is needed to answer those questions. Meanwhile, we suggest you speak to your healthcare provider if you have any questions about positioning your baby for sleep. Do not worry about back positioning interfering with the establishment of healthy sleep patterns. We have not found any indications that it does. .

DIAPERS, HYGIENE AND RASHES

Given the sensitivity of a newborn's skin, it's crucial to use water and a clean cloth. If you opt for commercial wipes, ensure they are specifically designed for newborns. Regardless of your choice, the wipes should be gentle, free from alcohol and perfume, to keep your baby's skin healthy and happy.

When cleaning your baby, always work from front to back (never back to front), especially on girls, to prevent the spread of bacteria that can cause urinary tract infections. Pay attention to the creases in the thighs and buttocks. For boys, a good practice to develop is holding a clean diaper over their genitals because exposure to air often causes boys to urinate with no regard for who is in the line of fire!

Diaper rash is a common concern and can be caused by various factors, from yeast infections to food allergies. If your baby has sensitive skin, they may be more prone to diaper rash. However, you can take proactive steps to prevent it by keeping your baby's skin dry and clean, changing diapers as often as needed, and avoiding prolonged exposure to urine and other excrement.

Most diaper rashes vanish in a few days with proper attention and over-the-counter creams. Check the labels for side effects if your baby is on any medication. If a rash persists, visit your healthcare provider for professional diagnosis and treatment.

FEVERS AND SICKNESS IN NEWBORNS

If your newborn shows signs of sickness or has a fever above 100.4° F /38° C, contact your pediatrician immediately. A fever in a young baby is of great concern to pediatricians. It can indicate a wide variety of infections—ear, bladder, kidney, or lung, perhaps—that only a professional can pinpoint. Although a fever is a sign that your baby's immune system is fighting off an infection, please stay mindful that a baby's immune system is not fully engaged until three months, leaving newborns more vulnerable to disease. Sickness and fevers are a natural part of life, and fortunately, we live in a time when most common bacterial and viral infections can be easily treated.

GRANDPARENTS

There is a special relationship between the third generation and the first. Within reason, you will want to take advantage of every opportunity for grandparents to enjoy your child. However, please do not assume your parents want to baby sit and do not abuse their generous offers. Above all else, do not surrender your parenting responsibilities to your parents. While they may enjoy their grandchildren very much and probably have a few good opinions about parenting, you are not the parents. We suggest you provide grandparents with their own copy of *Babywise Sleep Solutions* so they know what you are doing and why. That way, your baby will have a team on his side!

Here, we leave a message for Dad: Your role in managing the grandparents' visit is crucial. Many grandparents travel a great distance when the big day arrives. Of course, there is excitement and great anticipation, but that visit can either be a blessing or a problem, depending on your relationship with them and how like-minded they are with you. You might request that they postpone their visit until a few days or a week after the baby comes. By then, you will have worked through your basic parenting routine and feel familiar with it. Having a high-powered, take-charge relative come in right after birth is very hard on a new mother's emotions. Dad, your proactive approach can help protect your wife from that kind of stress and manage the situation for everyone's benefit.

IMMUNIZATIONS

The ability to protect children from the tragedies of many infectious diseases, such as Polio, Diphtheria, and Measles, is one of the great blessings of our day. To bring this blessing into your home, ensure your children receive all their recommended immunizations and receive them on time. Because immunization schedules change frequently as better vaccines become available, routinely ask your pediatrician for a current timetable of vaccinations for your child from now through college. The latest recommendations at this writing from the Centers for Disease Control and Prevention for infants include:

Hepatitis B vaccine
Rotavirus vaccine
Diphtheria and Tetanus Toxoids and Acellular Pertussis
    Vaccine (DPT)
Haemophilus influenza type b
Pneumococcal vaccine
Inactivated poliovirus vaccine
Influenza vaccine (seasonal)
Measles, mumps, and rubella vaccine (MMR)
Varicella (chickenpox) vaccine
Hepatitis A vaccine

While the Internet is a valuable resource for health information, many websites contain false and misleading information about the safety of vaccines. Consult your baby's pediatrician if you have questions about vaccines and immunization in general, but please get your children vaccinated!

MICROWAVE AND THE BOTTLE
For babies receiving formula, Mom or Dad will often rely on the microwave to heat the formula. A couple of cautions to mention. First, loosen the top of the bottle to allow for heat expansion so it does not literally explode. Second, beware that microwaves tend to heat food unevenly, creating hot spots, so shake the bottle well after heating and squirt a dab of milk on your wrist to test the heat level for warmth. A simple precaution but necessary.

Since excessive heat can destroy the nutrient quality of expressed breastmilk, we recommend that you avoid using the microwave to thaw or heat it. Instead, place the bottle of expressed breastmilk in a bowl or small pan of warm water.

Whether your baby is getting breastmilk or formula, most will take a bottle at some point. It is essential to keep the bottles and nipples clean and sterilized. There are bottle sterilizers designed to work in a microwave. These speciality items are available in a variety of models and price ranges. A dishwasher can do the job with cages that hold the nipples and other small items, but only if you tend to wipe your dishes and utensils visibly clean before loading them (that is, you do not treat your dishwasher like a garbage disposal). It helps to shake down the bottles and other items that retain water when the rinse cycle stops, so they dry properly during your dishwasher's drying phase.

NURSING TWINS

The *Parent-Directed Feeding* philosophy is an excellent friend to parents of multiples, especially in giving helpful advice about breastfeeding. Our experienced moms of twins find it best to assign a breast to each baby, and to keep them nursing on that specified breast throughout all feedings. This will help your milk supply keep up with the unique demand of each twin. Let one twin set the pace and keep them both on that schedule. If that means you must wake one, do so.

During the first few weeks post-partum, you can nurse your twins simultaneously using a football hold—arms bent to support the back and head of each baby while they nurse. As they grow, your babies will have to nurse one at a time. Beyond that distinction, you will be able to implement all other aspects of the *PDF* plan, including feeding routines and sleeping through the night.

Parents expecting multiples will find an entire section dealing with the practical management of multiples at *www.Childwise.Life*. Please take advantage of these resources.

PACIFIERS AND THUMB-SUCKING

There are many good reasons for using a pacifier with your newborn. It can help satisfy a baby's non-nutritive sucking need; it is soothing and can preempt periods of stress; and it is useful when Mom needs a few more minutes before she can get to the baby for a feeding. Furthermore, research suggests pacifiers may help reduce the risk of SIDS.

There are, however, a few warnings. First, the pacifier should not be introduced too early if Mom is breastfeeding. There is the possibility that the Baby might prefer the pacifier over the Mom because nursing requires more energy. Second, since the pacifier is a source of pleasure, it can become addictive. For example, a baby may depend on it to fall asleep or fall back asleep if waking early from a nap. Early on, the pacifier can be a parent's friend, but stay mindful that it does not become Mom and Dad's foe in six to eight months.

Children—infants, pretoddlers, and toddlers—suck thumbs and fingers out of habit more out of than a deep-seated psychological need for comfort. Infants find thumb-sucking soothing during times of stress, fatigue, or calm. Unlike the pacifier, the thumb is physically attached to the child, and the child can become habitually attached to the thumb. The good news is that 50 percent of infants give up thumb-sucking on their own by six to seven months of age. If either thumb-sucking or the pacifier becomes a problem after this period, you will find solutions spelled out in book two of this series.

PREMATURE BIRTH

While the average full-term gestation period is 40 weeks, a baby born from 37 weeks on is still considered full-term. Babies born before the 37th completed weeks of pregnancy are considered premature. In the 1980s, the rate of premature births fell to 3-5 percent. Today, that rate is approaching 13 percent. There are two explanations for this sharp rise: the number of multiple births has increased from advancements made with in-vitro fertilization, and the advances in obstetrics and neonatology have improved the chances of survival for even the smallest babies, even those born as early as 24 weeks after conception.

Thanks to medical science, babies born at 24 weeks have a 60 percent chance of survival. At 26 weeks, survival rates jump to 86 percent. Preemies that reach 32 weeks have a 99 percent chance of survival and a very low risk of health and development complications.

While most premature babies are at risk for some health problems, the closer to full term the baby is born, the less risk there is of severe complications. Size is also an issue for the premature infant. A baby born at 32 weeks will be significantly smaller than a baby at 40 weeks. That causes feeding challenges because preemies are sluggish eaters and can only take small amounts of food. Pediatricians who specialize in high-risk premature births usually recommend calorie and vitamin-enriched formulas or fortifiers to be added to breastmilk.

Since premature births are not planned, being aware of the possibility and understanding the risks will help any parent cope with the unexpected. Many reputable medical websites provide up-to-date information and the opportunity to ask questions related to premature births.

POSTPARTUM DEPRESSION (PPD)

Until your Baby is sleeping at least 6 hours or more during the night, Mothers usually fight some level of fatigue. However, if you find that after your six-week postpartum check-up, you are experiencing strong mood swings, have difficulty accomplishing minimal household tasks, or are constantly on the verge of tears during the day, please talk to your obstetrician. This state of mind and level of emotions at this point is not normal and is a symptom of postpartum depression (PPD). The phone call to your doctor is free, but the cost to yourself and the rest of your family is more than you probably will want to emotionally pay if you do not get help.

There are three levels of postpartum hormonal imbalance. The first and least serious level, the *Baby Blues*, is something most women experience right after birth. It usually peaks around the fourth or fifth day postpartum and typically disappears within ten days to two weeks. Moms experiencing the baby blues tend to cry over the most minor incidents, feel overwhelmed, lose concentration, and have difficulty sleeping. Unlike postpartum depression, baby blues is not an isolated condition. It can share the stage with Mom's feelings of joy, excitement, and happiness.

The second level of hormonal imbalance is Postpartum Depression (PPD), which can be set in a few days or even weeks after birth and is considered by healthcare authorities to be a more serious condition than a simple case of baby blues. Mothers experiencing PPD have feelings of depression, sadness, hopelessness, despair, and fatigue. They are often anxious, irritable, weepy, and unable to concentrate, and they can experience sleep and eating imbalances. A mother can greatly minimize the symptoms of PPD by keeping herself and her Baby on a good routine, which allows her to get quality rest and proper nutrition.

If she finds she is still abnormally melancholy after several weeks, she should seek counsel from her obstetrician.

The third level of imbalance linked to childbirth is Postpartum Psychosis. This is by far the most severe emotional state since it usually causes a break from reality. Symptoms include hallucinations, delusions, suicidal or homicidal thoughts, and disorganized thinking. A mother who has been previously treated with bipolar disorder is more likely to develop postpartum psychosis. Moms who suffer from this should see a physician as soon as possible. One in every 1,000 women who give birth suffers from this condition. This is no small matter, and the condition should be viewed with a sense of urgency.

STARTING SOLID FOODS

Introducing solid foods into a baby's diet does not mean stopping liquid feedings. The calories gained from breastmilk or formula are still of prime importance, but now your baby has reached a growth point where liquid feedings alone are no longer nutritionally sufficient.

Typically, babies start on solid foods between four to six months. While the AAP suggests waiting until six months, your pediatrician will provide personalized guidance based on your baby's nutritional requirements. There are specific developmental signs to watch for before introducing solids, such as your baby being able to control their neck and head muscles and sit upright (with support).

Other readiness indicators include your baby showing signs of hunger even though he receives 32 ounces of formula a day. If breastfeeding, he shows signs of hunger after 6-8 full feedings in 24 hours. The baby with a well-established nighttime sleep pattern and then between 16-24 weeks begins to wake at night or early during well-established naps, which may also signal that he needs more nutrition.

SWADDLING A BABY

Most newborns find comfort in the age-old practice of swaddling. This simple technique, which we encourage, helps to calm and comfort a fussy baby, facilitates sleep, and minimizes the startle reflex. Learning how to swaddle a baby is a straightforward process that any parent can master. All you need is a regular receiving blanket or a swaddle blanket. We offer a few cautions here. Be careful not to swaddle the baby too tightly since that restricts breathing and circulation, and be careful that the blanket does not cover the baby's face. There will come a time when your baby no longer enjoys being swaddled, and I will let you know. Just follow your baby's lead on this.

TEETHING

Teething is the term used when a tooth begins to break through the gum. It is all part of normal growth and usually starts between five and seven months. Generally, the lower two teeth come first, followed by the upper and middle teeth. Teeth tend to erupt sooner in girls than boys, but around two years of age, both boys and girls have, or are close to having, all 20 of their baby teeth.

Teething should not interfere with breastfeeding since the sucking reflex used while nursing is done by the tongue and palate, not the gums. Discomfort, irritability, fussiness, increased salivation, and a slightly raised temperature might accompany the eruption of a tooth but should not change your baby's feeding routine. You may find that teething causes a mild disruption to your baby's sleep but this too is temporary and will not override a well-established sleep pattern.

Your child should see a dentist around the time his first tooth comes into his mouth, but at the very least, make sure your child sees a dentist for a well-baby dental check-up by his first birthday. This is very important because early evaluation and education are the keys to preventing childhood dental diseases. Your dentist can help you determine your child's risk for tooth decay and help you with techniques to clean his teeth effectively and safely. Starting to visit the dentist at an early age helps your child become comfortable in a dental office. .

WEANING YOUR BABY

Weaning is the process by which parents offer food supplements in place of or in addition to mother's milk. That process begins the moment parents offer the first food supplement. From that moment on, weaning is a gradual process. As it relates to breastfeeding, there is no set age at which weaning is best or preferable.

When ready, a breastfeeding mom can start the weaning process by eliminating one feeding at a time, going three to four days before dropping the next one. This flexible time frame allows Mom's body to make the proper adjustments in milk reduction. Usually, the late-afternoon feeding is the easiest one to drop since it is a busy time of day. Replace each feeding with 6-8 ounces of formula or milk, depending on the child's age. (Pediatricians generally recommend babies not receive whole milk (cow's milk) until they are at least one year old.)

While Baby may not wean from the breast or bottle before his first birthday, Mom must think ahead by introducing the "sippy cup" around six to seven months of age. *Babywise Transitions* covers the practical side of this feeding option.

For the formula-fed baby, transitioning from the bottle to the sippy cup can start around 10-11 months of age. When you begin to wean from the bottle, start with the Noon meal. A few days later, eliminate the morning and late afternoon bottles. The evening bottle will be the last to go. This process takes time, so it's important to be prepared and patient, understanding that every baby is different and will adjust at their own pace.

With additional articles, books, research, and Babywise Mom feedback, we are constantly updating our *www.Childwise.Life* resource center. Please come visit.

Chapter Nine

What To Expect And When

One of the great parenting myths of our day is that parents will intuitively know what to do upon the arrival of their baby. In truth, first-time parents are apt to be stressed as they learn to adjust to the overwhelming presence of a helpless infant in the home. After leaving the security of the hospital staff, those first few days and weeks are likely to be filled with uncertainty.

It may not be possible to be fully prepared as a first-time parent, because along with the arrival of the first child comes a variety of new experiences and emotions. We do believe, however, that parents are better prepared to deal with the changes a baby brings to their lives when Mom and Dad have a basic understanding of what to expect in the days following birth. This Appendix describes what usually takes place during the first three days through the first three weeks after delivery. Becoming familiar with the various expectations will spare Mom and Dad unnecessary concern.

Next to each item listed, we provide two boxes to check. As you initially read through the list before your baby arrives, place a check mark (✓) next to each item in the first row of boxes. When you have a newborn sleeping in the next room, go through the list again and check the second box. Why two boxes? Because the first time you are reading to become familiar with the subject matter, but the second time you will have a burning desire to comprehend what if presented, driven by a heightened sensitivity for the welfare of a little life totally dependent on you.

WHAT TO EXPECT DURING DAYS: 1-3

☐ ☐ A baby is most alert right after delivery and usually ready to nurse.

☐ ☐ Colostrum is a baby's first milk and present at birth.

☐ ☐ After a Cesarean birth, Baby is usually able to nurse soon after Mom is moved to the recovery room.

☐ ☐ Baby's meconium stool (dark and sticky like tar) should have passed within the first 48 hours after delivery, followed by transition stools over the next several days.

☐ ☐ A baby should urinate within the first 24 hours after delivery.

☐ ☐ Within 24-48 hours, your baby should start having wet diapers, increasing to three to five per day as Mom's milk comes in.

☐ ☐ Babies usually lose 7-8 ounces from their recorded birth weight within the first 24-36 hours. Your baby's hospital-discharge weight is more reflective of your baby's actual body weight and is the better base line for your baby's growth.

☐ ☐ One of the biggest challenges of the first 72 hours is a baby's sleepiness. Parents must keep their baby awake to take full feedings approximately every 2-3 hours.

☐ ☐ Follow proper umbilical-cord care and hygiene at each diaper change. If your son has been circumcised, provide the appropriate care at each diaper change.

☐ ☐ In these early days, be more concerned with providing your baby 8-10 good feedings every 24 hours than establishing your baby's routine or sleeping patterns.

☐ ☐ Remember that for now, your baby's feeding time is his wake-time.

WHAT CONCERNS TO LOOK FOR: DAY 1-3

☐ ☐ The color of Baby's skin is yellow: After the first day, newborns usually develop jaundice, which produces a yellowish hue to their skin. If that happens, a doctor will usually order a blood test to measure the level of bilirubin, which then determines the course of treatment. If the yellow tint appears after discharge from the hospital, be sure to contact your baby's doctor.

☐ ☐ Baby is lethargic, very sleepy or unwilling to feed: While it is common for newborns in the first week to be sleepy, it should not interfere with feeding. If you are breastfeeding, make sure your baby is properly positioned at the breast and properly latched on. Seek the experience of a lactation consultant or your doctor if you have any concerns.

WHAT TO EXPECT DURING WEEKS: 1-3

☐ ☐ The transition milk comes in between days three and five and by week three, mature breastmilk should be in.

☐ ☐ Continue to focus on full feedings.

☐ ☐ Monitor your baby's growth using the Healthy Baby Growth Chart. By week two, the baby should have regained his birth weight or be close to it. (Download free copies from *www.Childwise.Life*.)

☐ ☐ The baby's stools will transition in color and consistency after the third day.

☐ ☐ The stools of breastfed babies tend to be softer and a lighter color than that of formula-fed babies. By five and seven days of age, a baby should have at least 3 to 5 loose yellow stools per day.

☐ ☐ By five to seven days, a baby should have a least 6-8 wet diapers, some saturated. Urine varies in color from nearly clear to dark yellow.

☐ ☐ Like adults, the color of the urine helps determine if your baby is receiving enough milk to keep him adequately hydrated. Colorless or pale-yellow urine suggests adequate hydration; darker, apple-juice-colored urine (by the end of the first week) suggests that Baby is not receiving enough milk.

☐ ☐ Continue providing umbilical-cord care at each diaper change until cord stump falls off. That usually happens around week two. During this time, the baby needs only a sponge bath: do not immerse him in water. Remember, if your son has been circumcised, provide the proper care with each diaper change until the circumcision is healed.

☐ ☐ Between ten days to three weeks, babies may have a growth spurt and require additional feedings. This may last from one to three days.

    ☐ ☐ For a breastfed baby, feeding could be as often as every two hours (possibly extending through the night) for one to three days.

    ☐ ☐ For a formula-fed infant, parents will notice that their baby appears hungry after consuming the normally-prepared number of ounces; or he is showing signs of hunger sooner than the next scheduled feeding. There are a couple of options to consider:

        ☐ ☐ Add 1-2 ounces to his bottle at each feeding, allowing baby to take as much as he wants. If baby was taking 2½ oz. per feeding, make a full 4 oz. bottle and allow him to eat until full; or

        ☐ ☐ Offer the extra feeding as Baby shows signs of hunger. When the growth spurt is over Baby will return to his normal feed-wake-sleep routine. However, on the day following a growth spurt most babies take longer than normal naps.

☐ ☐ By week three, alertness should be increasing at feeding times. Between weeks three and four, your baby's waketime will begin to emerge as a separate activity apart from eating. His schedule should look something like this: feeding, burping and diaper change takes about 30+ minutes. A little bit of waketime adds another 20+ minutes. Naptime is 1½ to 2 hours.

☐ ☐ Not all feed-wake-sleep cycles during the day will be exactly the same length of time. That is why a range of times is provided and not *fixed* times.

☐ ☐ If breastfeeding, do not allow your baby to go longer than 3 hours between feedings during the first three weeks. The feed-sleep cycle should not exceed 3 to 3½ hours during the first three weeks. At night, do not allow your newborn to go more than 4 hours between feedings. (Normal feeding times usually fall between 2½ to 3 hours.)

WHAT CONCERNS TO LOOK FOR: WEEKS 1-3

☐ ☐ By 5-7 days, if your baby is not having a least 6-8 wet diapers, or not having at least 3-5 loose yellow stools per day, contact your baby's pediatrician.

☐ ☐ Baby is unwilling to feed.

    ☐ ☐ If breastfeeding, make sure Baby is properly positioned at the breast, is latching on properly and that milk is being let-down. Check inside your baby's mouth for any presence of oral thrush, which is caused by the yeast Candida Albican. Signs include a milky white substance that coats the roof and side of the baby's mouth.

    ☐ ☐ If bottle feeding, make sure the nipple opening is neither too small nor too big. If too small, then Baby is sucking too hard to get the milk and may pull away. If the nipple opening is too big, the milk will come out too fast, usually causing Baby to gag and pull away. Change to appropriate size nipple.

☐ ☐ If your baby cries excessively before, during or after feedings, or if he is sleeping less than one hour and wakes up crying, call your pediatrician. Make sure you are keeping track of Baby's intake and output with the Healthy Baby Growth Chart,

There is so much more to learn and enjoy in the journey ahead. Visit us online to continue the dialogue at *www.Childwise.Life*. This is a great resource for our parenting journey.

Chapter Ten

Monitoring Your Baby's Growth

One of the many advantages of *parent-directed feeding* is the success mothers have with breastfeeding. Knowing your baby's nutritional needs are being met in an orderly fashion provides greater confidence with the overall parenting experience. However, a warning is necessary. While confidence is a positive thing, do not become complacent when it comes to monitoring your baby's growth.

This is important to us and should be to you. Your baby's life depends on it! Understanding what to expect in the first week and recognizing the nutritional signs to watch for can be a game-changer for your confidence and your baby's well-being. These signs offer Mom with direction and feedback on their progress. They affirm that things are on track and they alert of any issue that requires immediate attention. If you notice any unhealthy signs, it's crucial to contact your pediatrician immediately and share your observations.

On the *Childwise.Life* website the reader will find are age-related *Healthy Baby Growth Charts*, designed to assist you in your daily evaluation. These charts are free and easily downloadable The first Growth Chart is specifically to week one of your baby's life. The second chart covers weeks two through four, and the third chart covers weeks five and beyond. Using these charts will provide important benchmarks signaling healthy or unhealthy growth patterns.

What are the indicators that Mom and Dad should be looking for? Let's review them.

WEEK ONE: HEALTHY GROWTH INDICATORS

1. Under normal circumstances, it takes only a few minutes for your baby to adjust to life outside the womb. His eyes will open, and he will begin to seek food. Bring your baby to the breast as soon as it is possible, and certainly try to do so within the first hour and a half after birth. One of the first and most basic positive indicators is your baby's willingness and desire to nurse.

2. It is natural to wonder and even to be a little anxious during the first few postpartum days. How do you know if your baby is getting enough food to live on? The release of the first milk, colostrum, is a second important encouraging indicator. In the simplest terms, colostrum is a protein concentrate ideally suited for your baby's nutritional and health needs. One of the many benefits of colostrum is its effect on your baby's first bowel movement. It helps trigger the passage of the meconium, your baby's first stool. Newborn stools in the first-week transition from the meconium stool to a brownie-batter transition stool to a mustard-yellow stool. The three to five soft or liquid yellow stools by the fourth or fifth day are totally breastmilk stools and a healthy sign that your baby is getting enough nutrition. A bottle-fed baby will pass firmer, light brown to golden or clay-colored stools that have an odor similar to adult stools.

3. During the first week, frequent nursing is necessary for two reasons: first, your baby needs the colostrum and second, frequent nursing is required to establish lactation. Nursing every 2½ to 3-hours and a minimum of eight times a day are two more positive indicators to consider .

4. Just bringing your baby to the breast does not mean your baby is nursing efficiently. There is a time element involved. In those early days, most babies nurse between 30 and 45 minutes. If your baby is sluggish or sleepy all the time or does not nurse for more than ten minutes, this may be an unhealthy indicator.

5. As your baby works at taking the colostrum, you will hear him swallow. A typical pattern is suck, suck, suck, then swallow. When mature milk becomes available, your baby responds with a rhythmic suck, swallow, suck, swallow, suck, swallow. You should not hear a clicking sound nor see dimpled cheeks. A clicking sound and dimpled cheeks during nursing are two indicators that your baby is not sucking efficiently. He is sucking his tongue, not the breast. Remove the baby from the breast if you hear clicking, and then relatch him. When relatching, wait for your baby to present a wide open mouth. Look for lips to be flared out like fish lips. Use a finger to curl out the top lip if needed gently. Try gentle downward pressure on the baby's chin to draw out the bottom lip. If it is not resolved with practice, have it checked by a lactation consultant or your pediatrician. (This could be a potential tongue or lip tie.)

Week One Healthy Growth Indicators

1. Your baby goes to the breast and nurses.
2. Your baby is nursing a minimum of eight times in 24-hour.
3. Your baby is nursing over fifteen minutes at each nursing period.
4. You can hear your baby swallowing milk.
5. Your baby has passed his first stool called meconium. (Since the passage of the meconium is one of the "well baby" markers of a newborn, most hospitals will not release a baby if this stool has not passed within the first 24 hours. Failure to pass the meconium stool may signal an intestinal obstruction.)
6. Your baby's stooling pattern progresses from meconium (greenish black) to brownie batter transition stools to yellow stools by the fourth or fifth day. An increased stooling pattern is a positive sign your baby is getting enough milk.
7. Within 24-48 hours, your baby starts having wet diapers increasing each day to five to six by day five.

Unhealthy Growth Indicators for Week One

1. Your baby is not showing any desire to nurse or has a very weak suck.

2. Your baby fails to nurse eight times in a 24-hour period.
3. Your baby tires quickly at the breast and cannot sustain at least fifteen minutes at the breast.
4. Your baby continually falls asleep at the breast before taking a full feeding.
5. You hear a clicking sound accompanied by dimpled cheeks during nursing.
6. Your baby's stooling pattern is not progressing to yellow stools within a week's time.
7. Your baby has not produced a wet any diapers within 24 hours of birth.

WEEKS TWO - FOUR: HEALTHY GROWTH INDICATORS
After the first week, some of the healthy growth indicators begin to change. Here is the checklist for the next three weeks.

Healthy Growth Indicators for Weeks Two through Four
1. Your baby is nursing at least eight times a day.
2. Your baby has two to five or more yellow stools daily during the next three weeks. (This number will probably decrease after the first month.)
3. Your baby should start to have six to eight wet diapers a day (some saturated).
4. Your baby's urine is clear (not yellow).
5. Your baby has a strong suck, you see milk on the corners of his mouth, and you can hear an audible swallow.
6. You are noticing increased signs of alertness during your baby's waketime.
7. Your baby is gaining weight and growing in length. We recommend your baby be weighed within a week or two after birth. Baby should regain birth weight by day fourteen.

Unhealthy Indicators for Weeks Two through Four
1. Your baby is not getting taking eight feedings a day.
2. Your baby stools are small, scant, and infrequent.

3. Your baby does not have the appropriate amount of wet diapers.
4. Your baby's urine is concentrated and bright yellow.
5. Your baby has a weak or nonproductive suck, or you cannot hear him swallowing.
6. Your baby is sluggish or slow to respond to stimulus and does not sleep between feedings.
7. Your baby is not gaining weight or growing in length. Your doctor will direct you in the best strategy to correct this problem.

WEEKS FIVE AND ABOVE: HEALTHY GROWTH INDICATORS
The major difference between the first-month indicators and the weeks to follow are the stooling patterns. After the first month, your baby's stooling pattern will change. He may pass only one large stool a day or as infrequently as one every three to five days. Every baby is different. Any concerns regarding elimination should be directed to your pediatrician.

Parents are responsible for seeing that their baby's health and nutritional needs are recognized and met. For your peace of mind and your baby's health, we recommend regular visits with your pediatrician and use of the Growth Charts to monitor and record your baby's progress. Any two consecutive days of deviation from what is listed as normal should be reported to your pediatrician or health-care provider.

Download additional Healthy Baby Growth Charts from _www. Childwise.Life_

Appendix A

Right Beginnings

Most people are born into families where they inherit a way of living, a rhythm, a pulse that shapes the meaning of their existence. Home, for many, is more than a simple memory of a place where childhood unfolded. It is the first structure in which one encounters life, in all its complexity, its joys and fears, its quiet rituals. We learn it instinctively, through the everyday gestures of those who raised us.

The word "home" is dense with unspoken weight, steeped in the early breath of belonging. It permeates everything, especially in that first, delicate year, when the boundaries of our being are still forming, vulnerable to every influence around us. Nothing in life shapes a person more than the quiet, steady presence of a mother and father. Their influence is like a pulse in the walls of that home, undeniable, shaping who we become in ways we may not fully understand until years later. No other relationship reaches so deep or lingers as long as that between parent and child.

However, with that depth comes a testing ground—a place where personalities clash, resolve is tested, and the essence of one's self is measured against the needs of another. What are the silent burdens of parenthood? What questions must those expecting a child ask themselves in the lonely hours before birth? And more importantly, what beliefs must they cling to or let go of as they prepare for the weight of this irreversible commitment?

Although parenting is personal, it is still linked to larger truths.

There are certain beliefs about babies, about care and nurturing, that serve as beacons, guiding us through the fog of new parenthood. And yet, there are others—beliefs we must unflinchingly reject—if we are to give a child the sturdy, unshakable foundation on which to build their life, their heart, their mind..

The Challenge

Too often, couples step into parenthood with a quiet, unspoken hope that a sudden clarity will arrive, without their needing to prepare or understand the realities of raising a child. Even when they have taken classes, read books, or sought advice, the shock that comes with a newborn is still overwhelming. They find themselves disoriented, as if all the structures they once knew have crumbled, replaced by this small, demanding being whose needs alter the very fabric of their lives.

For the mother, this shift is felt in both her body and her heart. No longer connected to the child through the unseen, protective bond of pregnancy, she must now learn how to respond to an endless series of new signals—cries, gestures, tiny movements. These sounds will awaken emotions she didn't know she possessed, stirring her with an intense, almost primal urge to nurture, to protect, to sustain. The sense of responsibility is unlike anything she has ever experienced before, yet it is strangely familiar, as if she was always meant to feel this way.

For the father, too, the world shifts. He must now share his partner, his closest companion, with this fragile new presence. It is a quiet sacrifice, an unspoken trade—he gives up a piece of her attention, her time, and her warmth, only to receive something larger in return, the growth of their bond into something new and far-reaching. But this change, while profound, also extends beyond the emotional. It seeps into the small, daily details. Time, once free and fluid, now demands structure. The spontaneous moments that defined their relationship, the unplanned nights out or lazy Sundays, are gone. Everything becomes tied to the question, "What about the baby?"

Life shifts. It will never return to what it was, and this is where the true challenge lies. Some parents enter with the mistaken belief that life will continue as before, perhaps with only slight modifications. They imagine they will somehow keep the rhythm of their pre-child lives, only to be faced with the undeniable reality that nothing will be the same. Yet, it is equally false to assume that life will dissolve into chaos, that the quiet intimacy they once shared will vanish forever.

Change is inevitable. With a baby, it becomes the pulse of daily life. The success of navigating these changes, the ability to thrive in the midst of them, depends not on clinging to old patterns, but on understanding what this new life requires—both in the small moments and the grander scheme. It is this awareness, this willingness to adapt, that will shape the path forward..

WHAT'S MISSING?

We have seen many couples step into parenthood with bright eyes and open hearts, filled with hope and the promise of love, only to find their dreams unravel into a blur of exhaustion, desperation, and survival. Who are they? They are like anyone, perhaps like you—ordinary mothers and fathers. The couple you smiled at in your birthing class, the family whose stroller passes by your window each morning, or the neighbors with the cheerful stork sign on their lawn, wrapped in pink ribbons to celebrate the arrival of baby Alexis.

These parents, full of goodwill, come armed with an array of baby knowledge—facts and tips from books, advice from relatives—but something is missing. They possess the information, but not the understanding. Facts can fill pages, but it is understanding that gives them shape, makes sense of the chaos, and weaves them into a meaningful narrative. What is understanding? And why does it matter?

Understanding is more than knowledge; it is what transforms a series of isolated moments into a coherent, forward-moving path. It stretches beyond the immediate, casting its gaze toward the future. To parent with understanding is to see beyond the sleepless nights and crying fits. It is to recognize that each day builds on the last, that each small act of care links together—today with tomorrow, a week with a month, a year with a childhood.

This type of understanding is a compass, guiding parents through the twists and turns of raising a child. It minimizes confusion, allowing for fewer missteps along the way, and provides the clarity necessary to make decisions not just in the moment, but with the future in mind. The goal of this book is to offer new and expectant parents that deep sense of understanding—one that brings confidence to mothers and fathers and instills a lasting sense of security in their child.

The Impact on Children

Unlike animals, humans carry within them a unique strand of emotional DNA, one that refuses to be content with mere physical closeness in a marriage. It is this deep need for emotional connection, for a shared sense of being, that sets us apart. When a husband and wife are not unified—emotionally, physically, socially—there are gaps, fissures in the relationship. These gaps, though often invisible at first, can ripple outwards, affecting not only the couple but also their children.

A husband or wife might find ways to cope with the missing parts, to navigate around the voids. But children, especially babies, have no such defenses. They cannot rationalize or intellectualize their way through instability. They reach out with their senses, absorbing the world through touch, sound, sight, the smallest vibrations of their parents' emotions. This is why the love between a mother and father cannot be overstated: it is a kind of invisible glue, saturating the child's world with a sense of safety, security, and belonging.

Why does this matter? There is something almost magical about the love a child observes between their parents. It shapes their brain, their neural wiring, in ways that researchers are only beginning to understand. It is not the mother-child bond alone that predicts a child's future emotional security or intellectual success; it is what the child sees in the connection between their mother and father that holds the greatest weight. From the earliest days of life, children instinctively use their parents' relationship as a measure of the world's safety. If they sense harmony, the child's brain leans into growth, into exploration. But if the child detects even the faintest tremor of instability, the brain shifts, diverting energy away from growth and toward survival.[1]

The love within a marriage offers children something deeper than any direct parent-child relationship can provide, even in infancy. It is a kind of protective layer, a quiet assurance that allows the child to thrive. When all these elements come together—emotional unity, stability, love—they form the foundation of a home where a baby can flourish, where the brain can grow and reach for the future without fear.

The Warning

Too often, parents lose their way, or perhaps they never truly saw it to begin with. They become absorbed in the day-to-day wonders of parenthood—capturing photos, celebrating first steps and words. The baby becomes the center of their world, and slowly, the marriage fades into the background. For a time, this shift might feel natural, even joyous, for both mother and father. But in truth, it is not what the child needs most. The greatest gift parents can offer their child is not found in the isolated roles of mother or father, but in the unity they share as husband and wife.

Think about it. When the marriage is whole, when it is filled with beauty and tenderness, what child wouldn't be drawn into its warmth? When two people are united, their bond becomes a source of comfort, a place of refuge for the child. Parents teach their children the meaning of love not only through their direct actions, but through the quiet, steady presence of their relationship. It is in the way they look at one another, the small gestures of care that weave through the fabric of daily life.

Healthy parenting flows from a healthy marriage. It is from this shared foundation that true security and love emerge. Protect your marriage. Nurture it. For in doing so, you are safeguarding the very heart of your family.

MEETING EVERYONE'S NEEDS
What must parents understand to keep their marriages alive and thriving, ensuring that their influence as partners and parents is at its strongest? A few guiding principles may helps:

1. *Keep living!* Life does not stop with the arrival of a baby, though it may slow and change shape for a time. But even as you step into the roles of mother and father, you remain a daughter, a son, a sibling,

and a friend. The relationships that mattered before the baby was born still matter now, and they deserve to be nourished. Invite those who were part of your life before the baby—grandparents, friends—into your home when you are ready, as life begins to settle.

2. *Date your spouse.* If you had a habit of date nights before your baby was born, continue it when you can. If not, perhaps now is the perfect time to start. These moments don't need to be extravagant or long, but they are essential in keeping your marriage alive. And a strong marriage is the foundation of a healthy, emotionally secure family.

3. *Continue those loving gestures that were enjoyed before the baby arrived.* Whatever gestures once marked your relationship as special—those simple activities or gifts that brought joy—find space for them even after the baby arrives. If Dad brings home something for the baby, perhaps a small gift for Mom, too? The idea is simple: the love that made your marriage unique before parenthood should remain intact, sustained and nurtured throughout your journey as parents.

4. *Practice Couch Time.* At the close of the workday, take 15 minutes to sit together and talk about your day in front of your children. Amazingly, this small act provides children a clear, reassuring signal of Mom and Dad's emotional togetherness. By doing this, you help satisfy a longing within your child that continually seeks to know that all things are good between the two people I love the most—Mom and Dad! Couch Time becomes a visual cue, a symbol of stability and safety for the child. The more a child senses harmony in Mom and Dad's relationship the more emotionally secure the child becomes.

5. *Know what to expect of each other before your baby arrives.* The early days at home with a newborn are often the hardest—everything is new, overwhelming, unfolding at a pace you can't always control.

Couples typically settle into rhythms of shared responsibilities during pregnancy, but what happens after the baby is born? Those first cries, unfamiliar sounds, and the challenges of feeding and sleep will affect both of you in ways you haven't experienced before. Add postpartum emotions to the mix, and the first few weeks can quickly become a storm of stress.

To help minimize the stress a baby can bring into a normal home, parents should take the time to work through their expectations of each other, before their baby is born. Each person should know what household activity or chore he or she will be responsible for. Who will take care of the laundry and meals, shopping, vacuuming, furniture dusting, and who will get up to get the baby for the middle-of-the-night feeding? On the *Childwise.Life* website, the reader will find a convenient downloadable *"Who Will do What?"* check list. This simple list can save a lot of heart ache, frustration and tension after Baby arrives. This may seem like an insignificant to-do list right now, but we assure you, these common household chores are not so insignificant after the baby arrives.

A WORD TO THE SINGLE PARENT

Life, with its inevitable twists and turns, often veers us away from the idea, or what we think is the ideal. In the home, the ideal is to parent from the strength of a partnership, anchored in a marriage because two will always be better than one. But we know that this ideal is not the reality for everyone. The death of a spouse, the end of a marriage, or an unplanned pregnancy can shatter the dreams we once held, leaving us adrift in discouragement.

Having worked alongside single parents for over thirty years, we have come to understand the weight they carry—the constant demands of nurturing a child while also shouldering the roles of homemaker, provider, and protector. It is an exhausting dance, a balance that asks for more than seems humanly possible.

Yet, we also know this: if you are a single parent, you will love your baby with a depth no different than that of any couple. You will long to offer your child the best life you can, to protect them, to guide them, to nurture them. And it is our privilege to support you, to help you harness all your emotional and intellectual strength, no matter your circumstances.

If you are a single parent, know that while you may sometimes feel like an outsider in spaces designed for traditional families, in the realm of caring for your child, you are always, and will always be, welcome in our community. You belong here.

TO THE POINT

In parenting, everything is connected: the beginning with the end and everything in between. That means parents never act in any given moment without their actions having some impact on the future. That is true not just in the role of a mom or dad, but also as a wife or husband. As we have endeavored to point out throughout this book, every parenting decision will have a corresponding ripple effects that connect our beliefs and assumptions with our actions, and our actions with outcomes.

Keeping your marriage strong has positive consequences and therefore we encourage you to parent from the strength of your marriage and you will parent well. If you're interested in additional resources to strengthen your marriage, please visit our online resource center at *Childwise.Life*. This is a good place to connect with new and experienced *Babywise* moms.

Appendix B

Babywise Sleep Solutions Resource Page

The Supplemental resource pages serve as quiet companion to the various topics within the main text and points the reader to a network of online resources, that expands the discussion. There, the reader will find are articles, worksheets, and answers to questions, and some friendly voices who can walk you through those moments when a little encouragement might be needed.

The *Babywise Sleep Solutions* resource page can be accessed in two ways. For readers of the digital edition, a simple tap takes them directly to the additional content, offering instant access to a network of online resources. Paperback readers, on the other hand, must visit the *www. Childwise.Life* website to reach the same wealth of information.

Childwise.Life

The topics listed below are only a few of the many free supplemental aids and presented to provide the reader with a sense of confidence and direction while navigating through the landscape of early parenthood.

Relating to Breastfeeding:

Taking Care of Mom and Baby
This resource covers a newborn's development and growth characteristics that health care professionals will be looking for, as well as the physical and emotional challenges a mother might face postpartum.

The more expectant parents understand the changes that will be taking place after the baby arrives, the better prepared they will be when even the unexpected happens. While this resource may not be an urgent need, it is nonetheless an important one.

Who Will Do What? Checklist
For new parents, those first several days at home with a new baby are the most difficult because everything is new and unfolding. To help minimize the stress a baby can bring into a normal home, parents should take the time to work through their expectations of each other before their baby is born. Each person should know what household activity or chore they will be responsible for. Who will take care of the laundry and meals, shopping, vacuuming, and dusting, and who will get up to get the baby for the middle-of-the-night feeding? If you fail to define who will do what after the baby comes, then mom or dad will be at the mercy of the habits created by their in-laws, and for some, that could be a scary thought. Take some time to review each item on the *Who Will Do What?* checklist before the baby comes.

Colic, Reflux, and the Inconsolable Baby
One of the most significant medical risks associated with colic is not the condition itself but its symptoms since they mimic and often mask serious conditions such as milk-protein allergies, lactose intolerance, gastroesophageal reflux (GER), and gastroesophageal reflux disease (GERD). This chapter addresses three medical conditions. While each condition has its own diagnosis, they are related symptomatically through crying and spitting up. The three conditions explained include:

1. Colic
2. Gastroesophageal reflux (GER)
3. Gastroesophageal reflux disease (GERD)

Monitoring Your Baby's Growth (Charts)
One of the many advantages of parent-directed feeding is mothers'

success with breastfeeding. Knowing your baby's nutritional needs are being met in an orderly provides greater confidence. While confidence is positive, do not become complacent when monitoring your baby's growth. Knowing what to expect in the first week and what nutritional indicators to look for can make all the difference regarding your confidence and your baby's welfare. These indicators confirm that things are going well and warn of any condition that needs immediate attention. Call your pediatrician and report your objective findings whenever you notice unhealthy indicators.

Growth Expectations Week by Week
We believe parents are better prepared to deal with the changes a baby brings to their lives when Mom and Dad have a basic understanding of what to expect in the days following birth. This Appendix describes what usually takes place during the first three days through the first three weeks after delivery. Becoming familiar with the various expectations will spare Mom and Dad unnecessary concern.

Multiple Births
How to put the *Parent Directed Feeding* approach into practice with multiples.

Managing Your Baby's Day
Sample Schedules For Weeks 23-39 and Weeks 40-52

Expanded Waketimes and Nap Challenges Section
This includes charts, question and answers, and how to solve your baby's waking early challenges.

Problem-Solving
Here we explore the most common questions asked relating to the implementation of *PDF* strategy throughout Baby's first year.

Sleep Deprivation and Infants
Sleep deprivation has a profound impact on *myelination*, the process by

which the myelin sheath—a protective, insulating layer—forms around nerve fibers (axons) in the brain. When sleep is insufficient, several detrimental effects on myelination occur. Read about it.

Chapter Endnotes

Chapter One

1. Marc Weissbluth, Healthy Sleep Habits, Happy Child (New York, Ballantine Books 1987), p. 44.

Chapter Two

1. Journal of Human Lactation Volume 14, Number 2, June 1998, p. 101

Chapter Three

1. This conclusion was drawn from a study based on 32 mother-infant pairs observed over two years. Sixteen families were from the La Leche League, and the other sixteen were not. "Sleep-Wake Patterns of Breast-Fed Infants in the First Two Years of Life," Pediatrics 77, no. 3, (March 1986): p. 328.

2. American Academy of Pediatrics, "Does Bed Sharing Affect the Risk of SIDS?" Pediatrics 100, no. 2 (August 1997): p. 727. (Update July 2022)

3. American Academy of Pediatric Policy Statement, Pediatrics, Vol. 116 no. 5 November 2005, p. 1247.

Chapter Six

1. Pediatrics, 100, no. 6 (December 1997): p. 1036.

2. Ibid., p. 1036

3. Sources supporting these recommended number of feeding times: American Academy of Pediatrics Policy Statement Pediatrics 100, no. 6, (December 1997): 1037; Frank Oski, M.D., Principles and Practice of Pediatrics, 2nd ed. (Philadelphia: J.B. Lippincott Company,

1994), p. 307; Richard E. Behrman, M.D., Victor C. Vaughan, M.D., Waldo E. Nelson, M.D., Nelsons Textbook of Pediatrics, 13th ed. (Philadelphia: W.B. Saunders Company, 1987), p. 124; Kathleen Huggins, The Nursing Mother's Companion, 3rd ed. (Boston: The Harvard Common Press, 1995), p. 35; Jan Riordan and Kathleen Auerbach, Breastfeeding and Human Lactation, (Sudbury, MA.: Jones and Bartlett Publishers, 1993), pp. 188, 189, 246.

4. Breastfeeding mothers are sometimes warned not to use a bottle. The concern is over "nipple confusion." The belief is that a baby will become confused and refuse the breast if offered a bottle. Although under normal circumstances there will be no need to introduce a bottle to the breast-fed infant in the first few weeks, there will come a time when the bottle will be a welcome friend. After the first few days of breastfeeding, supplementing by bottle rarely causes "nipple confusion." Kathleen Huggins, The Nursing Mother's Companion, 3rd ed. (Boston: Harvard Common Press, 1995), p. 73.

Chapter Seven

1. Caring for Your Baby and Young Child—Birth to Age Five: The Complete and Authoritative Guide (The American Academy of Pediatrics), ed. Steven P. Shelov M.D., F.A.A.P. (New York: Bantam Books, 1998), pp. 34-47.

2. Study cited by Mary Howell, M.D. in baby! Vol. 2 No.2. The Healthy Baby 1987, p. 27.

3. Ibid., p. 189.

4. Ibid., pp. 188-89.

5. Ibid., pp. 36.

Chapter Eight

1. Michael E. Lamb, Ph.D., from the Department of Pediatrics at the University of Utah Medical School, summarizes our position: "The preponderance of the evidence thus suggests that extended contact [the bonding theory] has no clear effects on maternal behavior." Michael E. Lamb, Ph.D., in Pediatrics, 70, no. 5 (November 1982), p. 768.

2. For an excellent challenge to the myth of bonding, please see Diane Eyer, Mother Infant-Bonding: Scientific Fiction, (New Haven: Yale University Press. 1992).

3. Pediatrics (August 1997), p. 272.

Appendix A

1. See the collaborating work of Dr. John Medina. Dr. Medina is a developmental molecular biologist specializing in the genes involved in human brain development. He is the author of the Brain Rules and Brain Rules for Baby. (Pear Press 2010)

Subject Index